Pass the MRCPsych Essay

W.B. Saunders Company Ltd
24–28 Oval Road
London NW1 7DX

The Curtis Center
Independence Square West
Philadelphia, PA 19106–3399, USA

Harcourt Brace & Company
55 Horner Avenue
Toronto, Ontario M8Z 4X6, Canada

Harcourt Brace & Company, Australia
30–52 Smidmore Street
Marrickville, NSW 2204, Australia

Harcourt Brace & Company, Japan
Ichibancho Central Building, 22–1 Ichibancho
Chiyoda-ku, Tokyo 102, Japan

A catalogue record for this book is available from the British Library

ISBN 0–7020–2154–7

Typeset by Keystroke, Jacaranda Lodge, Wolverhampton
Printed and bound in Great Britain by WBC, Bridgend, Mid. Glamorgan

Pass the MRCPsych Essay

Edited by

Christopher Williams
Peter Trigwell

W.B. Saunders Company Ltd
London   Philadelphia   Toronto   Sydney   Tokyo

Contents

Contributors   vi

Foreword   *Professor A.C.P. Sims*   viii

Preface   x

1. Essay technique   1

2. Treatment resistant depression   13

3. Treatment resistant schizophrenia   25

4. Cognitive behaviour therapy   41

5. The treatment of eating disorders   65

6. Difficult issues in liaison psychiatry   89

7. Practical child psychiatry (within a child mental health team)   115

8. Molecular genetics in psychiatry   141

9. Personality disorder   165

10. Community care   185

11. Issues in transcultural psychiatry   201

12. Setting up and auditing an old age psychiatry service   229

Index   243

Contributors

Dr Nick Brindle BSc(Hons), MBChB, MRCP, MRCPsych
Wellcome Research Fellow, Molecular Medicine Unit, St James's University Hospital, Beckett Street, Leeds LS9 7TF

Dr Chris Buller BSc(Hons), MBBCH, MMedSc, MRCPsych
Senior Registrar in Adult Psychiatry, Airedale Hospital, Skipton Road, Steeton, Keighley, West Yorks BD20 6TD

Dr Stephen Curran BSc(Hons), MBChB, MRCPsych, MMedSc
Lecturer/Honorary Senior Registrar in Old Age Psychiatry, St James's University Hospital, Beckett Street, Leeds LS9 7TF

Dr David Hargreaves BSc, MBChB, MRCPsych
Senior Registrar in Forensic Psychiatry, Newton Lodge Regional Secure Unit, Ouchthorpe Lane, Wakefield WF1 3SP

Dr Christine M Hodgson-Nwaefulu BMedSci, BMBS, MRCPsych
Senior Registrar in Psychiatry, St James's University Hospital, Beckett Street, Leeds LS9 7TF

Dr Asma Humayun MBBS, MRCPsych
Senior Registrar in Psychiatry, St James's University Hospital, Beckett Street, Leeds LS9 7TF

Dr Peter Trigwell MB, ChB, MMedSci, MRCPsych
Senior Registrar in Psychiatry, Department of Liaison Psychiatry, Leeds General Infirmary, Great George Street, Leeds LS1 3EX

Dr Chris Williams, BSc(Hons), MBChB, MMedSc, MRCPsych
Lecturer/Honorary Senior Registrar in Psychiatry, Clinical Sciences Building, St James's University Hospital, Beckett Street, Leeds LS9 7TF

Dr Simon Wilson, BMedSci(Hons), BM, BS, DCH
Tutor/Registrar in Psychiatry, Malham House Day Hospital, 25 Hyde Terrace, Leeds LS2 9LN

Dr Barry Wright, MBBS, MRCGP, MRCPsych, DCH, MMedSc
Consultant in Child and Adolescent Psychiatry, Lime Trees Child and Adolescent Unit, 31 Shipton Road, York YO3 6RE

Dr David Yeomans BSc, MB ChB, MMedSc, MRCPsych
Consultant Psychiatrist, Somerset House, Manor Lane, Shipley, West Yorkshire BD18 3BP

Foreword

Professor A.C.P. Sims

A straw poll of MRCPsych examiners, not meticulously conducted in its methodology, concluded that most MRCPsych essays are marked between 9 p.m. and 12 midnight, with quite a few in the hour or two either side of that, while others are marked at the weekend. Clearly, it is a challenge for the examiner to stay alert, to remain marking with the same standard throughout and to ensure an adequate level of discrimination between the very good and very bad. It is even more of a challenge for the examination candidate to stand out from the amorphous mass for reasons of excellence rather than a horrible error or erratic howler! To do this the candidate has to argue logically, defend a case knowledgeably and, if possible, even interest the examiner.

The essay is not a test of memory; if we, as psychiatrists, wanted to assess our trainees' memories, we would test them with "digit span" or "name and address at 3 minutes". It is not primarily a test of knowledge. The MRCPsych essay is a practical exercise in arguing the case, showing that one's thinking in terms of attitudes and skills and knowledge is that of a professional, trained psychiatrist. **Essay** means "try" or "attempt"; as examiners we are looking for a good attempt, a well-scored try.

Why read (or write) a book on what is after all only a rite of passage, passing a professional examination? Writing a good psychiatric essay can be more valuable than just passing the examination so that the appropriate letters can be placed after the successful candidate's name. The essay is an attempt to argue the case convincingly, a skill which will have career-long benefits for writing letters to general practitioners, preparing reports on behalf of patients for the Court, constructing research papers or case histories for professional journals and meetings, and even defending one's clinical practice to sceptical management or incriminating lawyers.

A few years ago, as President of the Royal College of Psychiatrists, I wanted to be informed (with more than just statistical data) about unusual topics of relevance to mental health care; I instituted the President's Essay Prize to do just that – for my own benefit. An essay gives the opportunity to create a literary, rhetorical and educational gem. Unfortunately, the MRCPsych essay often falls far short of that!

I am sure that the readers of this book will find it helpful and informative at the most prosaic level of simply passing the examination. However, there is more to it than that. The authors convey their own enthusiasms and give practical ideas and suggestions so that essay writing might even become enjoyable beyond the narrow examination context. The chapters of this book, on many different topics (which are outlines for essays in themselves), set a standard that could not be attained under examination conditions. However, if they are worked through carefully they will establish correct habits for improving both form and content. The approach is to craft a reasoned discourse that has itself been prepared before the examination, rather than to plonk a dollop of incomprehensible and indigestible "word salad" on the hapless examiner's plate! Careful reading of this book is likely not only to improve the candidate's mark in the MRCPsych essay, but also to produce long-term benefits in presenting professional information and opinion.

Andrew Sims, Professor of Psychiatry, University of Leeds.
Immediate Past President of the Royal College of Psychiatrists.
March 1996

Preface

There have been recent changes to the MRCPsych examination structure. One of the most important is in the essay paper for Part II of the MRCPsych. In the past, the candidate was required to choose one essay to answer from a list of six. This format has now changed. From Autumn 1995, the candidate must choose **two essays from a list of four**. They must answer one general adult psychiatry question out of two and one "sub-speciality" question out of two. In the past, it was usually possible to avoid certain subjects which the candidate particularly disliked when the choice was "one from six". With the new "two from four" system this will no longer be possible.

There are certain topics which lend themselves well to the essay question format. Some involve "high profile" clinical topics or are areas of controversy. Because of this they are increasingly likely to appear on the essay paper in forthcoming exams. These topics are often those which are not covered well from any one source (textbooks, journals, clinical experience, etc.), and so are particularly difficult to learn for essay purposes. This book summarises a range of these important topics in a structured, easy to learn form, in addition to giving clear advice on essay technique. It is hoped that candidates will also find the information useful in other parts of the MRCPsych examinations.

We are grateful to all the contributors, and also to Dr S. Lally and Professor A. C. P. Sims for their contributions to the book. We would also like to thank Alison and Amanda for their encouragement and support.

Chris Williams, Peter Trigwell
August 1996

Chapter 1

Essay technique

David Yeomans

When did you last write an essay? If like many exam candidates you have not written an essay for years, this chapter should help revive forgotten skills and provide you with some techniques for exam success.

The essay is not negatively marked, but you will still need to demonstrate a factual and accurate understanding of the question. Furthermore, you must present that account in good English using correct spelling and grammar. Your essay needs a **structure** and will benefit from a lively writing style. Your examiner, after marking several essays which are meandering and tedious, may well be tired and irritable. You need to make your essay the exception; a legible and interesting piece of prose.

Preparation

When you draw up your revision timetable be sure to set aside regular time to practice essays. Writing is physically tiring and is a skill which you may not have practised for several years. By the end of your revision you should have written **10–20 essay plans and at least two full length pieces**.

Reading is your major source of factual information. Textbooks plus revision books will give you enough factual material to pass, but additional material from specialist books, journals, clinical experience and conferences will increase your chances. You cannot read everything, so be selective. Review articles in major journals (e.g. *British Journal of Psychiatry*) and review journals (e.g. *Current Opinion*) are useful. Read the exam syllabus in the *Inceptor's Handbook* (from Royal College of Psychiatrists) to see which areas you need to know and which you do not. Send off for past papers and obtain the most recent exam papers from colleagues who have recently taken the exam.

Essay Spotting

There are several assumptions underlying the technique of essay spotting:

- Certain topics are important and these tend to be repeated.

- If such a topic has not come up recently then the chances of it appearing as a question in the next exam (your exam) are increased.

- Currently topical issues are often set on the essay paper (e.g. nation-wide changes in service provision, Mental Health Act, prominent review articles). Look at the editorials and reviews which have appeared in the last 12 months of the *Psychiatric Bulletin* and the *British Journal of Psychiatry*.

- Work out what major topics you wish to cover. Many candidates find it useful to produce a collection of "essay plans". If you prepare several topics, at least some of them may be included in whole or part form in the actual exam.

Structure

What is an essay?

- It is a long written piece held together by a **structure** and contains **arguments** supported by **information**.

- A common structure for an essay is an **introduction**, then the **arguments**, followed by your **conclusion**. This may need to be modified depending on how the essay question is asked. A very open question such as *"Describe the uses of medical audit"* requires you to define the structure yourself. A question such as *"Discuss the effects of antidepressants on the course and outcome of anxiety disorders"* is more clearly defined, but you must still impose some structure upon your answer.

Your answer can be structured using the following techniques:

- **Six useful questions** are: *"Who? What? Why? Where? When? How?"*. When tackling the essay ask yourself these questions to help produce a critical discussion. Think about what terms the question uses. *What* is medical audit? *Who* is interested in audit? *Why* should doctors get involved? *How* is anxiety defined? *How many* different antidepressants are there? *What* is outcome? *How* is it measured?

- **Helicoptering** (Fig. 1.1). A helicopter can hover a long way up in the sky to obtain a **broad** view of the situation. It can descend to various points in that landscape to see **more details**. You can do this in an essay by focusing in and out, to offer both a

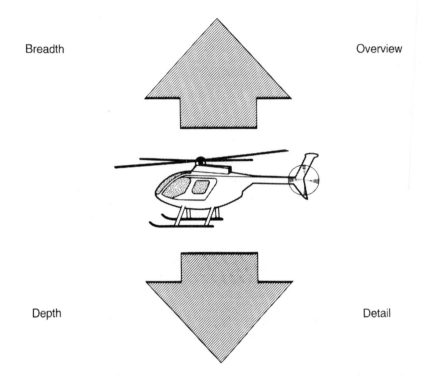

Breadth

Overview

Depth

Detail

Fig. 1.1 Helicoptering.

general overview and also specific detail and argument.

- **Expansion**. Before setting pen to paper expand the question to its limits by considering all the subject areas you can include. Helpful sub-headings to expand the scope of your thinking (and hence your essay) include:

  - Biological, psychological and social aspects.
  - Acute, intermediate and long term.
  - Male and female differences.
  - Age differences.
  - Cultural differences.

- "Non-medical" factors such as the impact on carers, media influences, politics and finance.
- Past, present and future implications.

Worked Example 1

Candidates on the Leeds MRCPsych Part II revision course were asked to use the above techniques to create essay plans. Although no one felt prepared for the task, one group produced the following essay structure within 10 minutes:

Question

"Discuss medical classification and how it has been applied in psychiatry".

Answer

Introduction, *"Why is classification necessary?"*:

- Communication.

- Universal use.

- Prediction of prognosis.

- It aids research so that different researchers can study similar patients.

- Implications for treatment.

Classification methods:

- Syndromal (grouping of symptoms and signs).

- Aetiology (infective, trauma, genetic, etc.).

- Course (acute, chronic or remitting).

- Outcome.

- Multiaxial definitions (or a combined biopsycho-social model).

Application of classification models in psychiatry:

- The current systems. ICD, DSM.

- Lack of success, lack of clear aetiologies and the limitations of syndromal classification.

- Outcome prediction is actually quite poor.

- Historical perspective, e.g. Kraepelin.

Conclusions:

- Slow but steady progress is being made.

- More consensus now exists than previously.

- Future hope is to include more aetiological and pathological data with multiaxial descriptions being taken into account.

The essay structure demonstrates some of the techniques previously described:

- First of all, you **must read the question in full**.

- A simple approach with an **introduction**, **arguments**, and **conclusion** is used.

- There is a **clear structure**. The candidates in this case **defined** *what* classification is and *why* it is used.

- They **helicoptered** down from the two broad questions on classification and application and split each up into several headings. For some of the headings they helicoptered down further to give detailed examples which illustrate the benefits and pitfalls of using diagnostic systems. They then helicoptered up again to allow a wider discussion of the arguments.

- The essay structure is **critical** and asks *how* successful classification is in psychiatry. It looks to *what* the future may hold and **expands** the question a little beyond what was asked.

- Perhaps it could have included some consideration of **cultural differences** and similarities. You may already have different ideas of how you would answer this question. Why not try them out now?

Worked Example 2

Question

"How can exploratory psychotherapy lead to a worsening of a patient's condition? What can be done to reduce this?"

Answer

Introduction – Definitions:

(a) **Exploratory psychotherapy**: dynamic psycho-therapy, types/methods; individual/group/family; in children and adults.

(b) **Worsening**:
  (i) In therapy – transference/counter transference issues, and risks of dependency.
  (ii) Out of therapy – acting out; also to consider problems in work or with their family.

(iii) General – risks of parasuicide/self-harm, anxiety or depression.

Arguments

This section could go on to discuss the above ideas, and particularly to discuss the "worsening" in terms of overall outcome.

What can be done to reduce worsening?

- Patient selection, including liaison with referrers.

- Training and supervision of psychotherapists.

- Conjoint work and treatment (e.g. additional medication from general practitioners).

- The importance of clear communication and continuity of treatment.

- Close monitoring of the mental state.

- Assessment of defence mechanisms for potential vulnerability to psychological treatment approaches.

- Attention to transference and countertransference issues and difficulties.

- Adequate preparation for times of absence by the therapist.

- Consideration of the frequency of sessions and the risks of dependency occurring.

The candidates' reaction to this essay title was interesting. Initially they felt great pessimism when given this question to attempt. They said that they would never have chosen this topic in an exam, and felt that they would answer it very badly because they did not have any specialised expertise in this field. None expected to produce such an extensive outline until they applied the techniques taught above. They were surprised to find out exactly how much they really knew. Had this been the only question they could remotely hope to answer, this technique-based approach would have given them more than a fighting chance of passing.

The Role of the Examiner

Pity the examiner who has to mark a lot of essays on the same question. Remember he or she may well be bored and miserable, sitting at home perhaps, with dogs barking and kids crying. It is your task to present them with a clearly legible, well written, structured essay that stands out from all the others.

What to Do

- Write legibly. **One examiner failed a candidate in 5 seconds because the essay was unreadable.**

- Consider writing double spaced. This makes your essay easier on the eye and simpler to mark. Break up the text with headings, lists, diagrams and tables where appropriate. (Take a look at your textbooks and see how they present information. Each chapter in the book is itself an essay.) Use colour (e.g. a red pen) to highlight important points or sub-headings using underlining.

When you sit the essay paper, spend a few minutes before you start writing to prepare an **essay plan**. Write out your essay structure at the beginning, on the exam paper, and label it as the "essay outline". You can then refer back to it as you write, in order to maintain the structure and keep track of the remaining time. Cross out those areas you have covered so that you can see how the essay is progressing. Take time to review the content intermittently in case any fresh ideas come to mind.

Write naturally, but consider the following. Short sentences add impact. Long sentences with no punctuation such as commas that go on for line after line and talk about different subjects without so much as a pause between them do tend to confuse and the examiner does not want to re-read the essay 10 times to work out what you are trying to say. See?

Show the examiners that you can order information, and make the presentation and structure clear by the use of sub-headings.

- Bullet points can be very effective in lists.

References need not be given in full. Names will usually suffice.

What Not to Do

Don't make things up. Don't waffle about irrelevancies. Do not write about a totally different question just because you have prepared an essay plan about it. You will get no marks unless you answer the question which is asked. Remember this point when you have spotted a question. You need to tailor the prepared answer to the question on the exam paper. Do not be unbalanced in your arguments. Remember that your essay reveals things about you. Examiners may be concerned if, for example, you appear to have no consideration for patients' well being. Finally, remember that an essay requires a reasonably lengthy piece of writing – one page is not enough!

What are your Blindspots?

When you write a practice essay, ask someone to comment critically about it. You may be unaware of habitual spelling or grammatical errors. You may not notice a tendency to leave words unfinished (the author has this proble). Let someone else discover your blindspots, but be critical of their criticism. In the end you have to rely on your own style.

Key points

- Practice writing full length essays.

- Prepare 10–20 outline essay plans using spotting techniques.

- Read the question carefully. Answer the question that is asked!

- Structure the essay plan using critical questions, helicoptering and expansion techniques. Write the essay plan down at the beginning of the exam and use it to pace yourself.

- Write legibly.

- Make your essay interesting and visually appealing.

Chapter 2

Treatment resistant depression

David Hargreaves

The frequency of this topic at case conferences indicates its importance as a difficult clinical problem. For essay purposes, however, it is well encapsulated and can be tackled in a systematic way. Consider the following.

Definitions

- Variable in the research literature[1] making comparisons of different studies difficult.

- Important to distinguish actual treatment resistance from mere chronicity of symptoms.

- A common **clinical definition** is failure to respond to adequate courses (high enough doses for long enough) of two antidepressants. Alternatively, failure to respond to an adequate course of one antidepressant and electroconvulsive therapy.

- An example of an "adequate course" would be a tricyclic antidepressant for 6 weeks at the maximum dose tolerated (within British National Formulary (BNF) guidelines).

Apparent Treatment Failure

This may result from:

- Incorrect diagnosis; i.e. it is **not** a depressive disorder.

- Inadequate initial treatment.

- Poor compliance; the patient is not taking the tablets.

- Incomplete formulation of the case – especially the role of maintaining factors.

- Co-morbidity.

The differential diagnosis for a possible depressive disorder includes:

Physical disorders:

- Endocrinopathies (e.g. hypothyroidism).

- Malignancy (e.g. occult cancer).

- Viral infection (e.g. influenza).

- Vitamin or other dietary deficiency (e.g. iron and vitamin B12).

- Drug side effects (e.g. nifedipine or steroids).

Psychiatric disorders:

- Anxiety disorders.

- Obsessional disorders.

- Post-traumatic stress disorder.

- Schizophrenia.

- Dementia.

- Alcohol/drug abuse.

- Eating disorders.

The presence of these disorders must be considered if depression does not improve.

Occasionally the treatment response may be partial, leaving a residue of resistant symptoms. Consider the possibility of "**double depression**".[2] Double depression is defined as a depressive illness superimposed upon longer-term dysthymia. This is unlikely if symptoms remain severe.

Risk Factors for Treatment Resistant Depression

This is an under-researched area. Factors such as concurrent medical illness and alcohol/drug abuse may be important. Personality disorders may be associated with a poor recovery in depression (see Chapter 9). Delays initiating treatment and higher premorbid neuroticism were found to predict persistence of symptoms in one study.[3]

Potential Consequences of Resistant Depression

- Loss of quality of life.

- Family break-up.

- Therapeutic alienation.

- Premature death – especially malignant and cardiovascular disease.

- Suicide.

- There is a significant economic impact on the individual, their family and their workplace in addition to costs to the State. The latter may include the costs to the Health Service (medication, out-patient and in-patient costs, psychotherapy referral, Community Psychiatric Nurse input, etc.) as well as to Social Services (including incapacity/invalidity and other benefits).

Pharmacological Treatments

Comprehensive reviews are available[4] as well as descriptions of practical management approaches,[5] and these should be consulted. Consider first the rationale behind ongoing pharmacological approaches. The basis of such approaches is to increase the availability/effective action of the monoamines noradrenaline and serotonin. With regard to serotonin this can be achieved by:

1. **Increasing precursor**: L-tryptophan is the precursor of 5-hydroxytryptrophan. Prescription of this amino acid has been shown to increase the levels of serotonin in the brain.

2. **Blocking re-uptake**:
    *   Tricyclic antidepressants (TCAs).
    *   Selective Serotonin Re-uptake Inhibitors (SSRIs).
    *   Serotonin Noradrenaline Re-uptake Inhibitor (SNRI – venlafaxine).

3. **Blocking degradation**:
    *   Monoamine Oxidase Inhibitors (MAOIs).
    *   Reversible Inhibitors of Monoamine Oxidase A (RIMA – moclobamide).

4. **Enhancing second messenger activity**: *lithium augmentation* has been shown to be an effective intervention,[6] and this may be used with tricyclic

antidepressants or, with caution, SSRIs (beware the "serotonin syndrome" – see below). Reports of very rapid response when added to tricyclics (within 48 hours) have been made.[7]

Serotonin syndrome

- Tremor at rest.
- Hypertonicity.
- Myoclonus.
- Autonomic signs.
- Hyperreflexia.
- Nystagmus.

Pharmacological approaches are only part of the management plan. An integrated treatment package that addresses physical, psychological and social aspects of care is essential.

A Practical Plan of Management

1. **Review of diagnostic formulation**:
   - Is the diagnosis of depressive disorder correct?
   - Are there any maintaining factors which need to be addressed (physical, psychological or social)?

2. **Check the patient's understanding of how to take the medication**: are they complying with the treatment?

3. **Continuation of monotherapy, and increase of dose to the limit of tolerability**:

   - Tricyclic antidepressants may, in some circumstances, be increased to 300 mg. Simpson et al.[8] showed 300 mg/day imipramine to be more effective than 150 mg.

   - The usefulness of monitoring plasma levels remains debatable, but has enthusiastic advocates in order to avoid toxicity.

   - The use of SSRIs in doses above maximal British National Formulary (BNF) limits is particularly to be avoided, due to lack of experience with these drugs.

4. **Change of medication**:

   - Switching to an alternative re-uptake inhibitor of the same drug group is unlikely to succeed once an adequate trial has failed, given the similar modes of action.

   - A change to a drug with a different mode of action can be effective e.g. an MAOI or RIMA may be a better choice, particularly if the clinical syndrome is "atypical" (with features such as anxiety, phobic symptoms, weight gain, hypersomnolence, etc.). Bear in mind the need for a washout period (see BNF guidelines; e.g. 5 weeks washout is necessary in the case of fluoxetine).

5. **Augmentation with a mood stabiliser**:

   - **Lithium** – prophylactic properties in bipolar and unipolar illness. It also acts as a weak antidepressant by increasing serotonin.

   - **Carbamazepine** – effective prophylactic agent but despite structural similarity to tricyclics lacks efficacy as an antidepressant. Avoid combination with tricyclics, since cytochrome P450 liver enzyme induction markedly reduces tricyclic levels.

6. **Other combination therapies**:

- **L-tryptophan** – no longer restricted to named patients. Case reports suggest effective in combination with lithium and clomipramine, or lithium and phenelzine (the so-called **"Newcastle cocktail"** developed by Eccleston). Can precipitate the serotonin syndrome – do not combine with selective serotonin re-uptake inhibitors. L-tryptophan is usually prescribed at 3 g/day. Previous problems with a myalgia–eosinophilia syndrome resulted from a contaminated production source. This has now been rectified.

- **Thyroid hormones** – in some cases, adding thyroxine to a tricyclic antidepressant may be useful even in the absence of clinical hypothyroidism.[9] Sub-clinical hypothyroidism has been implicated. May also have a role in rapid cycling illness.

- Other agents including sodium valproate and clonazepam have been suggested, but evidence regarding efficacy is lacking.

- **MAOI and tricyclic combination** – potential risks of serotonin syndrome and hypotension but some combinations (e.g. amitriptyline and phenelzine), appear safe. Start the tricyclic first or start both together. NEVER use clomipramine or tranylcypromine in combination.

- **SSRI and tricyclic combination** – increasing reports of use have appeared but the therapeutic rationale is difficult to justify. Potential problem of cardiotoxicity, as SSRIs (with possible exception of citalopram) are known to increase tricyclic levels. A review of 41 articles found "there is scant literature evidence to support the use of SSRIs in combination with TCAs as a treatment for refractory depression."[10]

- **Neuroleptics** – reduce psychotic symptoms irrespective of diagnosis.[11] They are therefore of proven effectiveness in psychotic depression. As with the SSRIs, they reduce tricyclic antidepressant metabolism, hence increasing antidepressant levels.

7. **Repeat courses of electroconvulsive therapy (ECT):** particularly if persistent biological or psychotic symptoms, or previous ECT was unilateral.

8. **Psychosurgery:**

- This may be vital for the small number of otherwise intractable cases. The risks of continued depression (weight loss, dehydration and infection, suicide, etc.) coupled with the extreme distress of continuing depression, means that psychosurgery should be considered.

- Informed consent **and** a second opinion is required (under section 57 of 1983 Mental Health Act – if in England or Wales). In addition, the psychiatrist must convince the Mental Health Act Commission that appropriate physical and psychological (e.g. behavioural and cognitive therapy) treatments have been adequately tried.

- Higher success rate if previous good social functioning, normal personality, previous history of treatment responsiveness, biological features and family support.

- Postoperative rehabilitation is very important, and improvement may be slow over months.

- 68% recovery rate for depression after sub-caudate tractotomy.[12]

9. **Other treatments**: Other treatments such as light therapy[13] and sleep deprivation[14] remain helpful in a few. Sleep deprivation may be useful as a diagnostic aid in depressive pseudo-dementia. The short-lived improvement that occurs in 60% of patients if they are kept awake overnight allows the psychiatrist to have an idea of the clinical improvement that is possible with effective antidepressant treatment.[15]

Remember that:

- Definitive evidence for the effectiveness of many of the above pharmacological interventions is lacking.

- Spontaneous remission remains a possibility. This reflects two processes:
  (i)   Regression towards the mean is the statistical likelihood that symptoms will improve.
  (ii) The natural "life" of a depressive illness is between 6 and 12 months without any treatment. Time itself may well lead to improvement in some.

- Psychological and social interventions remain important aspects of management.

The Role of Psychosocial Factors in Treatment

Always consider the role of maintaining factors including:

- Personality disorder.

- Alcohol or other psychiatric or physical co-morbidity.

- Chronic stressors such as work or relationship problems, debt, etc. Many patients feel like they do for a reason. Offer specific help for these.

- Specific psychotherapies have a role in treatment resistant depression. In particular, cognitive behaviour therapy has a useful role, even in bipolar disorder.[16]

Key points

- Depressive illness requires appropriate management from the outset – delays in treatment may predispose to chronicity.

- Treatment of resistant cases remains largely empirical, but a clear and justifiable rationale is possible.

- Always review the diagnosis and look for maintaining factors in resistant cases.

- Always consider physical, psychological and social factors.

- An awareness of important and potentially dangerous drug interactions is essential.

References

[1] Nierenberg A A, Amsterdam J D (1990). Treatment-resistant depression: definition and treatment approaches. *Journal of Clinical Psychology*, **51**, (Suppl 6), 39–47.

[2] Keller M B, Shapiro R W (1982). "Double depression": superimposition of acute depressive episodes on chronic depressive disorders. *American Journal of Psychiatry*, **139**, 438–442.

[3] Scott J Eccleston D, Boys R (1992). Can we predict the persistence of depression? *British Journal of Psychiatry*, **161**, 633–637.

[4] Nierenberg A A, White K (1990). What next?: a review of pharmacologic strategies for treatment resistant depression. *Psychopharmacology Bulletin*, **26**, 429–460.

[5] Bridges P K, Hodgkiss A D, Malizia A L. (1995). Practical management of treatment-resistant affective disorders. *British Journal of Hospital Medicine*, **54**, 501–506.

[6] Austin M P V, Souza F G M, Goodwin G M (1991). Lithium augmentation in antidepressant resistant patients. A quantitative analysis. *British Journal of Psychiatry*, **159**, 510–514.

[7] de Montigny C, Coumoyer G, Morisette R, Langlois R, Caille G (1983). Lithium carbonate addition in tricyclic antidepressant-resistant unipolar depression. *Archives of General Psychiatry*, **40**, 1227–1234.

[8] Simpson G M, Lees J H, Cuculic Z, Kellner R (1976). The dosages of imipramine in hospitalised endogenous and neurotic depressives. *Archives of General Psychiatry*, **33**, 1093–1102.

[9] Gupta S, Masand P, Tanquary J F (1991). Thyroid hormone supplementation of Fluoxetine in the treatment of major depression. *British Journal of Psychiatry*, **159**, 866–867.

[10] Taylor D (1995). Selective serotonin re-uptake inhibitors and tricyclic antidepressants in combination. Interactions and therapeutic uses. *British Journal of Psychiatry*, **167**, 575–580.

[11] Johnstone E C, Crow T J, Frith C D, Owens D G C (1988). The Northwick Park "functional" pscyhosis study: diagnosis and treatment response. *Lancet*, **11**, 119–124.

[12] Bartlett J, Bridges P, Kelly D (1981). Contemporary indications of psychosurgery. *British Journal of Psychiatry*, **138**, 507–511.

[13] Rosenthal N E, Sack D A, Gillin J C (1984). Seasonal affective disorder: a description of the syndrome and preliminary findings with light therapy. *Archives of General Psychiatry*, **41**, 72–80.

[14] Wu J C, Bunney W E (1990). The biological basis of an antidepressant response to sleep deprivation and relapse: review and hypotheses. *American Journal of Psychiatry*, **147**, 14–21.

[15] Williams C J, Yeomans J D I, Coughlan A K (1994). Sleep deprivation as a diagnostic instrument. *British Journal of Psychiatry*, **164**, 554–556.

[16] Scott J (1995). Psychotherapy for bipolar disorder. *British Journal of Psychiatry*, **167**, 581–588.

Chapter 3

Treatment resistant schizophrenia

Simon Wilson

Introduction

Following the initial treatment for a schizophrenic illness:

- 10–30% of patients will have residual psychotic symptoms.[1]

- Many patients will be handicapped by negative symptoms.

The effective management of these patients is a challenge to both the health services and the clinician. It requires a positive and optimistic approach, examining the breadth of the patients disabilities (and abilities). Even a small improvement in chronic symptoms can have a large impact on the lives of patients and relatives, and can help make the difference between coping with the illness and despair.

Definition

Treatment resistance is defined as a failure to achieve acceptable remission of positive symptoms despite an adequate trial of three different classes of antipsychotic, each given in adequate dosage for at least 6 weeks.[2]

Management of Treatment Resistant Schizophrenia

Management should follow a logical pattern and adopt a broad approach covering physical, psychological and social factors.

- Review the diagnosis.

- Review current treatment.

- Consider the range of physical, psychological and social interventions available.

Review diagnosis and current treatment

Review the history, mental state examination and treatment to date. Is the diagnosis correct? There are specific points you should consider in order to cover the possible psychiatric and organic differential diagnoses.

- **Affective illness**: consider whether there is a significant affective component to the illness presentation. Is it a "schizoaffective" disorder? If there is a significant affective component, either manic or depressive, specific drug treatment of this is warranted.

- **Organic delusional disorder**: undiagnosed organic illness, e.g. temporal lobe epilepsy, sarcoidosis with cerebral involvement, etc. may all cause a presentation that may be mistaken for schizophrenia.

- **Dual diagnosis**: for example, co-existent schizophrenia and alcohol or substance abuse. Up to

57% of patients with schizophrenia abuse illicit drugs or alcohol at some time.[3] Alcohol and drug abuse may worsen the psychotic presentation and cause treatment resistance.

- **Drug interactions**: anticholinergics reduce the effectiveness of neuroleptics.[4] It is important to remember this when procyclidine or other anticholinergics are prescribed. Other common medications such as cimetidine and carbamazepine accelerate the metabolism of haloperidol. Remember to check for possible drug interactions.

Review compliance

Poor compliance with medication occurs in up to 60% of out-patients and 30% of in-patients.[2] Consider factors which lead to poor compliance:

- Inadequate information – the patient does not understand the rationale for treatment.

- Difficult drug regimen – the patient is too disorganised and forgetful to be able to take their medication regularly.

- Poor insight and denial.

- Unwanted side effects.

Review for psychosocial stressors

Consider high **expressed emotion** in relatives which predicts frequent relapse.[5] The "emotional temperature" of the home environment is a potent predictor of the risk of relapse of schizophrenia. Read an up-to-date review of this field, such as the one by Kavannagh.[6] High expressed emotion refers to a number of components that are found during an interview made by the researcher with the family and carers of the patient. The interview is recorded and ratings are made for the following:

- Hostility.

- Critical comments.

- Emotional overinvolvement.

- Amount of contact per week (greater than 35 hours increases risk of relapse).

Investigations

(a) Physical

Consider the following investigations for each patient:

- Plasma viscosity.

- Syphilis serology.

- Plain chest X-ray.

- Urine drug screen.

- Electroencephalogram (EEG).

- Computerised tomography of the head.

(b) Psychosocial assessment

- Interview relatives and carers.

- Occupational therapy assessment.

- Social work assessment (benefits, housing and day centres).

- Discuss patient with the Community Psychiatric Nurse or named nurse.

- Liaise with GP.

Treatment Options

A broad-based approach with physical, psychological and social interventions is essential.

Physical interventions

Remember that the definition of treatment resistance requires failure of remission on three different antipsychotics for at least 6 weeks.

- Has the patient been treated for long enough to allow sufficient time for a response?

- Improvement with neuroleptic medication may continue for up to 12 weeks or more. Is your diagnosis of treatment resistance premature?

Consider the following strategies if the patient fulfils the criteria for treatment resistance:

(a) Altering the route of administration

There are wide variations in plasma levels of neuroleptics given by different routes,[7] so consider changing the route of administration.

(b) Altering the dose of neuroleptic

This may involve either increasing or decreasing the dose of neuroleptic.

- A lack of nursing staff on wards may lead to the inappropriate prescription of higher doses of neuroleptics.

- Polypharmacy with a range of neuroleptics prescribed concurrently is not recommended.

- Owing to adverse effects at high doses some patients may improve with a reduction in dose.

This acts to reduce possible drug neurotoxicity such as drug-induced akathisia, agitation and iatrogenic negative symptoms.

High dose neuroleptics

The dose may be increased up to British National Formulary (BNF) limits. There is little scientific evidence to support the effectiveness of increasing doses above these limits. Increased doses are accompanied by increasing side effects and risks of toxicity.

It is argued by some that higher dose neuroleptics may be required to overcome a lack of efficacy of pharmacological treatment when BNF recommended doses are used. Arguments made by those who support this policy include:

- Inadequate systemic concentration may occur as a result of idiosyncratic metabolism/elimination of the drug, thereby causing the lack of response. This is uncommon.

- Inadequate D2 blockade may be occurring. However, at doses of 15 mg of haloperidol or 400 mg of chlorpromazine there is a 75–80% block of D2 receptors in the basal ganglia on Positron Emission Tomography (PET) scans. Increasing the dose adds little to this dopamine blockade.

- D2 blockade may be limited to certain brain areas such as the basal ganglia; hence effective D2 blockade is not achieved where it really matters (i.e. in the mesolimbic system).

- Higher doses allow the blockade of additional important non-D2 receptors such as D4 and 5HT type 2 receptors.

Dangers of high doses of neuroleptics

- **Sudden death**. This occurs through a number of effects including profound hypotension, negative inotropism and dysrhythmias as a result of blockade of sodium and calcium channels. The risk of cardiac arrhythmias is increased and appears related to dose.

- **Extra-pyramidal side effects** are increased. It is important to consider the risk of irreversible tardive dyskinesia which may be increased by the use of long-term, high dose neuroleptics.

- Risk of **neuroleptic malignant syndrome** may be related to the rate of increase of dose.

- **Paradoxical violent behaviour** may occur as a result of atropinic effects, akathisia or as a withdrawal rebound reaction.

- General effects on the **central nervous system** (e.g. respiratory depression, seizures and coma).

Royal College Consensus statement[1]

This is an important document. You should obtain and read this:

- Doses higher than recommended by BNF should only be instigated by a consultant or post-membership psychiatrist. *"A junior psychiatrist (Senior House Officer or Registrar without MRCPsych) is not considered to be sufficiently qualified to take a decision to raise the dose of antipsychotics above the recommended upper limit. This applies particularly in the emergency and acute situation where junior doctors on call appear regularly to exceed BNF doses"*.

- *"Prescribing outside the (drug) licence alters and probably increases the doctor's professional responsibility"*.[8]

In general for high doses to be used the Consensus statement suggests:

- **Obtain consent**. Discuss with patient, family and multidisciplinary team. Record your decision and reasoning behind it in the notes. Consider obtaining a second opinion.

- **History**. Record an assessment of cardiac status, hepatic/renal function, weight, use of alcohol and tobacco, and age.

- If under Section, make sure there is compliance with **Part IV of the Mental Health Act** (1983).

- **Review other drugs**. There is increased risk of arrhythmias with tricyclic antidepressants, antihistamines and diuretics, or if the patient is suffering hypotension or abnormal urea and electrolytes.

- **Review ECG**. Watch for ST depression, inverted T waves and a prolonged QT interval. Repeat every 1–3 months. If a prolonged QT interval develops, reduce the dose and review.

- Carry out **regular observation** of pulse, blood pressure and temperature.

- **Urea and electrolytes** should be checked regularly.

- **Increase the dose in small steps**. Increases should occur at intervals longer than 1 week in order to adequately assess response.

- **Review progress**. Stop after 3 months if no response.

- All psychiatrists should have **experience in resuscitation**. An appropriate procedure for dealing with cardiac arrest should be developed in each hospital and ward.

(c) Atypical antipsychotic drugs

An atypical antipsychotic is **a neuroleptic which has a low propensity to produce extra-pyramidal side effects at clinically effective doses**. Examples include sulpiride, remoxipride, clozapine and risperidone.

Clozapine is licensed for use when two other neuroleptics have failed to give a response, or because of intolerance to neurological side effects such as tardive dyskinesia:

- In treatment resistant schizophrenia, there is a 30% response rate after 6 weeks treatment, and 54% response at 6 months in clinical trials.[9]

- Both positive and negative symptoms respond to clozapine and it has been shown to reduce aggressive behaviour and suicide attempts.

- Clozapine has a higher affinity for D1 and D4 receptors than classical antipsychotics but lower affinity for D2 receptors. It binds to 5HT type-2 receptors which may explain its atypical action.

- The most important (although rare) side effect of clozapine is agranulocytosis which occurs in 0.8% of patients after 1 year of treatment. As a result, all patients have to be registered with the manufacturer for regular blood tests.

- The Clozapine Patient Monitoring System (CPMS) requires the treatment to be instigated as an in-patient, and a weekly blood sample must be sent by post to the manufacturer. Other neuroleptics are tailed off as the dose of clozapine is increased. Depot medication must be stopped prior to starting clozapine, in case agranulocytosis develops.

- Blood tests are graded by the CPMS according to a "traffic light" system. A green light means that the drug supply will be released by pharmacy. An amber light means that closer attention must be paid to blood tests and clinical state as the white cell count has dropped a little. A red light means that treatment must be suspended and a medical opinion is sought.

- In cases of agranulocytosis, medical admission may be necessary.

- There is a continuing debate on the indications for using clozapine – mainly because of the high financial costs involved. In spite of the additional financial costs of the CPMS, its use has been advocated earlier in treatment for some patients due to its effects on negative symptoms and social functioning.[10]

- It seems likely that in the long term the use of clozapine saves money in some patients, with fewer admissions to hospital being necessary.

Risperidone is a new antipsychotic with few extra-pyramidal side effects. It is effective against both positive and negative symptoms. It is also said to be effective for the depressive symptoms which are often seen in the setting of a schizophrenic illness.

(d) Adjunctive drug treatments

- Benzodiazepines may be of benefit, particularly where anxiety is pronounced. There are risks of tolerance and dependency if taken on a regular basis.

- Propranolol can lessen autonomic symptoms of anxiety and akathisia.

- Lithium can improve psychotic symptoms in those patients with prominent affective symptoms.

(e) Electroconvulsive therapy

- Electroconvulsive therapy improves positive symptoms in some patients in the short term, especially when given together with neuroleptics. It may be useful where speed of recovery is important or **catatonic features** are present.

- In a double-blind trial, improvement with electro-convulsive therapy (ECT) at 4 weeks was not maintained at 12 weeks or 6 months. Thus, there is little evidence for the use of ECT in long-term management.[11]

Psychological interventions

(a) Supportive psychotherapy

There is a 15% suicide rate in schizophrenia. Maintaining a trusting long-term relationship with patients is essential. Patients at most risk of suicide are those who are young, male and intelligent. During both recovery and episodes of relapse these are the people who may feel the most hopeless and damaged by their illness. Deliberate self-harm and suicide may also accompany psychotic experiences or substance misuse.

(b) Social skills training

Poor social skills and antisocial behaviour can be modified by using a combination of operant behavioural techniques and other training.[9] Patients may role play social situations with a therapist who reinforces correct behaviour. A simpler educational programme may be helpful.

(c) Rehabilitation service referral

Specialist rehabilitation services with trained staff can offer a wide variety of interventions aimed at identifying the patients strengths and weaknesses. Specific work can be done looking at areas such as self-care, safety in the kitchen, and the ability to look after a house or flat. Many patients with resistant positive or negative symptoms will need help finding accommodation appropriate to their abilities and needs (e.g. their own flat, shared house, group home, warden accommodation or inpatient unit, etc.). Occupational therapy, training courses and paid employment are all important potential goals.

(d) Cognitive behaviour therapy

Patients are taught about the nature of their illness and origin of their symptoms through a trusting alliance with a therapist. They are taught to monitor psychotic symptoms and identify faulty reasoning. Patients are encouraged to see themselves as not intrinsically different from others (a "normalising" approach) and to question their delusional beliefs by planned reality testing.[12] Using techniques of problem solving and coping strategy enhancement in patients with neuroleptic resistant psychotic symptoms, significant improvements were reported in one controlled trial.[13]

Social interventions

(a) Intervention with families

Patients living with relatives where the relationship is characterised by high expressed emotion (i.e. hostility, emotional overinvolvement and/or frequent critical comments), are more likely to relapse than those living in a household of low expressed emotion. Living with a family of low expressed emotion is as valuable clinically as maintenance medication.

Controlled intervention studies to reduce expressed emotion show significant reduction in relapse rates over 2 years. Leff *et al.*[14] showed a reduction in relapse rate from 78% for those patients on depot medication alone to 14% in the intervention group. Interventions of value for families of high expressed emotion are:

- Education programme for relatives.

- Relatives support groups.

- Family sessions with the patient.

- Reducing face-to-face contact with relatives to less than 35 hours/week.

(b) Intervention in the community

For patients with a history of frequent relapse and poor compliance, regular contact with community support workers lessens social isolation and improves social functioning.[15] Even with effective community support the burden is heavy for carers. Mutual support groups for carers such as The National Schizophrenia Fellowship may help relieve a sense of isolation as well as provide practical advice and help.

(c) Care programme approach (CPA) and supervision registers

The enactment of community care legislation and closure of long-stay psychiatric beds means that most patients with treatment resistant schizophrenia will be managed in the community. The report by Ritchie *et al.*[16] into the care and treatment of Christopher Clunis has highlighted the importance of co-ordinated action between agencies involved in patient care, if patients with chronic mental illness are not to slip through the net. Patients with treatment resistant schizophrenia should be offered a care programme to include:

- A named care programme co-ordinator.

- An explicit care-plan.

- Assessment of their health and social needs, which

are then addressed in a planned and organised way.

- A date when their care is to be reviewed, of which others involved (including carers) are aware.

- Placement on the supervision register of those patients who are at risk of serious self-neglect, or of committing serious violence or suicide.

By using the whole range of physical, psychological and social interventions available for schizophrenia some patient's symptoms will improve. For those patients whose symptoms remain resistant to treatment, there can still be improvements in social functioning and quality of life.

Key points

- Treatment resistance is a failure to achieve acceptable remission of positive symptoms with three different classes of antipsychotic given at adequate dose for at least 6 weeks.

- Review the diagnosis and previous treatment considering the role of compliance and possible maintaining factors.

- Management should adopt a broad approach addressing physical, psychological and social aspects.

Physical interventions include:

- Change route or dose of neuroleptic.

- Atypical antipsychotics, e.g. clozapine, especially if extra-pyramidal side effects are troublesome.

- Adjunctive medication, e.g. lithium.

- Electroconvulsive therapy may have a role.

Psychological interventions:

- Supportive psychotherapy.

- Social skills training.

- Cognitive behaviour therapy.

Social interventions:

- Reduce high expressed emotion in families.

- Consider specialist occupational therapy or rehabilitation assessment.

- Regular social support and contact, e.g. day centre.

- Care programme approach (also consider supervision register).

References

[1] Thompson C (1994). Consensus statement Royal College of Psychiatrists. The use of high-dose antipsychotic medication. *British Journal of Psychiatry*, **164**, 448–458.

[2] Anon (1995). The drug treatment of patients with schizophrenia. *Drugs and Therapeutics Bulletin*, **33**: 81–86.

[3] Smith J, Hucker S. (1994). Schizophrenia and substance abuse. *British Journal of Psychiatry*, **165**, 13–21.

[4] Johnstone E C, Crow T J, Ferrier I N *et al*. (1983). Adverse effects of anticholinergic medication on positive schizophrenic symptoms. *Psychological Medicine*, **13**, 513–527.

[5] Vaughn C E, Leff J P (1976). Influence of family and social factors on the course of psychiatric illness. *British Journal of Psychiatry*, **129**, 125–137.

[6] Kavannagh D J (1992). Recent developments in expressed emotion and schizophrenia. *British Journal of Psychiatry*, **160**, 611–620.

[7] McCreadie R G, Mackie M, Wiles D H *et al*. (1984). Within individual variation in steady state plasma levels for different neuroleptics and prolactin. *British Journal of Psychiatry*, **144**, 625–629.

[8] Drugs and Therapeutics Bulletin (1992). Prescribing for unlicensed drugs or using drugs for unlicensed indications. *Drugs and Therapeutics Bulletin*, **30**, 97–99.

[9] Kane J M, McGlashan T H (1995). Treatment of schizophrenia. *Lancet*, **346**, 820–825.

[10] Kerwin R W (1994). The new atypical antipsychotics. *British Journal of Psychiatry*, **164**, 141–148.

[11] Brandon S, Cowley P, McDonald C *et al.* (1985). Leicester ECT trial: Results in schizophrenia. *British Journal of Psychiatry*, **146**, 177–183.

[12] Kingdon D, Turkington D, Carolyn J (1994). Cognitive behaviour therapy of schizophrenia: the amenability of delusions and hallucinations to reasoning. *British Journal of Psychiatry*, **164**, 581–587.

[13] Tarrier N, Beckett R, Harwood, S *et al.* (1993). A trial of two cognitive-behavioural methods of treating drug-resistant residual psychotic symptoms in schizophrenic patients: I. Outcome. *British Journal of Psychiatry*, **162**, 524–532.

[14] Leff J, Kuipers L, Berkowitz R *et al.* (1985). A controlled trial of social intervention in the families of schizophrenic patients: two year follow-up. *British Journal of Psychiatry*, **146**, 594–600.

[15] Thornicroft G, Breakey W R. (1991). The COSTAR programme. 1: Improving social networks of the long-term mentally ill. *British Journal of Psychiatry*, **159**, 245–249.

[16] Ritchie J H, Dick D, Lingham R (1994). *The Report of the Enquiry into the Care and Treatment of Christopher Clunis*. London: HMSO.

Chapter 4

Cognitive behaviour therapy

Chris Williams

Cognitive behaviour therapy (CBT) is recognised as an effective individual psychotherapy that may be used alone, or in combination with medication. It focuses on altering unhelpful thoughts or behaviours that may be contributing to the clinical problem.

Good outcome in controlled trials has been found in:

- Depressive illness.

- Generalised anxiety disorder.

- Panic attacks; probably the treatment of choice (up to 90% response rate).

- Bulimia; probably the treatment of choice.

- Obsessive compulsive disorder.

- Social phobia.

- Post-traumatic stress disorder (PTSD).

Key people historically include:

- **George Kelly**[1] who developed the **constructivist** cognitive therapies.

- **Albert Ellis**[2] who developed **rational emotive therapy** (RET).

- **Aaron T. Beck**[3] who developed **cognitive therapy** – now the most widely used approach.

Theoretical Basis

- What we believe affects our emotions and behaviour.

- When we are depressed or anxious our beliefs change characteristically by becoming:

    (i) **Inaccurate** with persistent cognitive errors. The beliefs often become exaggerated, distorted and untrue.

    (ii) **Unhelpful** – they worsen mood, alter behaviour and are potent maintaining factors for depression and anxiety, etc.

The theory does not state that the beliefs **cause** the illness, but rather that altering unhelpful beliefs may be an effective **treatment**. This does not involve positive thinking. Instead, the person is encouraged to try to **test out** whether their beliefs are accurate.

Predisposing factors

- Early childhood experience leads people to form **assumptions** or **schemas** (rules about **self/world/future**).

- Purpose of schemas is to organise perception/ evaluate behaviour and make sense of experience.

- Schemas may be helpful and adaptive, or unhelpful and maladaptive (dysfunctional).

- **Dysfunctional schemas** (untrue and unhelpful) are important in cognitive therapy.

Dysfunctional schemas/assumptions

These are inaccurate or unhelpful rules/beliefs which are:

- Rigid.
- Extreme.
- Resistant to change.

Typically they are **global beliefs** about:

- Self (e.g. *"I am bad/unlovable"*).
- The world (*"Unless I am loved by others, I am worthless"*).
- The **schema** may lie dormant and relatively inactive (or readily challenged or ignored) until external life events (**critical incidents**) activate the schema fully.
- The **critical incident** is often **a loss** in depression or **a threat** in anxiety, and this interacts potently with the particular schema held by the individual. Once activated, the schema comes to dominate thinking via **negative automatic thoughts** (NATs) and **cognitive distortions**. These then act to maintain the adverse mood change.

Negative automatic thoughts (or images):

- "Pop" into the mind.
- Are not based on reason.
- Are unpleasant.
- **In depression**, tend to revolve around themes such as worthlessness, guilt, incompetence, failure, and hopelessness. Negative predictions are made.

- **In anxiety**, cause the person to focus on catastrophic predictions that the very worst possible outcome will occur.

- Crowd out "rational" thoughts.

- Lead to a lowering of mood, increased anxiety, and/or altered behaviour.

- May be unrecognised by the person until they start to notice them as part of the treatment approach (e.g. by collecting information in thought diaries).

Cognitive Therapy Treatment Strategies

Selection of patients

- Patient acceptance of the model.

- Ability to make **thought–feeling** and **thought–behaviour** links.

- Form a relationship/work as a team with the therapist.

Traditionally, treatment has avoided psychotic or bipolar patients. These are now increasingly being seen as cognitive models are developed to help these patient groups (see Chapters 2 and 3).

Style of therapy

- Focuses on **changing unhelpful beliefs**.

- **Short-term/time limited** (normally up to 12–20 weekly sessions of 1 hour).

- **Structured and directive**. The therapist and client are active and collaborative, working together to establish goals.

- **Problem oriented**. Focused on problems maintaining difficulties rather than origins.

- **Collaborative empiricism**. Systematically **gathers evidence for and against** the client's beliefs in a manner akin to the scientific model of discovery.

- **Socratic questioning** is used to help the client make their own discoveries through **guided discovery**.

- View thoughts/beliefs as **hypotheses** to be tested (*"Are there any other ways of explaining that?"*).

- **Educational**. Skills and understanding need to be acquired.

- **Agenda setting**. Each session is planned for effective use of time and to provide a focus for treatment.

- **Use of homework tasks**. The client works on their problem on all days of the week, not just in the treatment settings.

- Use of rating scales to **monitor progress**/change.

- **Trying out strategies in session**: role-play or role-reversal to rehearse skills. Reviewing, and learning from the effectiveness of such strategies in homework assignments.

Education

Information about the condition: what depression or anxiety are, and how they affect thinking, the body and other symptoms.

Gathering information

- Self-monitoring.

- Diaries of thoughts/feelings in different situations.

- Generating **a list of problems** and formulating the case using the cognitive model.

Identifying thoughts from recent experiences

- Looking for situations that have led to sudden changes of mood (*"What went through your mind when your mood dropped?"*).

Challenging the automatic thoughts

- **Hypothesis testing**. Examining the **evidence for and against** the belief being true (*"It **may** be true that you have achieved nothing at all today, but shall we try and find out if that is the case?"*)

- **Hypothesis generation**: (*"Are there any other ways of explaining why she said that to you?"* – (e.g. she was late for work and trying to leave quickly).

- **Reality testing** (*"Why not **ask** her if she was bored by the conversation to find out if that is why she seemed to leave so quickly"*).

- **Behavioural tests/experiments**. Acting against the belief and seeing what happens, etc.

Teaching new skills

- Activity scheduling (decide to start doing things again in a planned and structured manner).

- Social skills training.

- Assertiveness training (learning to say no).

- Distraction techniques (so that they are not preoccupied by depressive thoughts).

- Relaxation skills.
- Problem solving.
- Time management.

The Cognitive Model of Depression

A critical incident (often a loss) leads to the activation of underlying schemas. This leads to characteristic changes in thinking which maintain the depression:[3]

1 **Beck's negative cognitive triad**. Negative views are held of:

 - Self.
 - Future.
 - World.

2 **Occurrence of cognitive distortions (thinking errors) (see Table 4.1)**. The activated schemas distort perception and memory so that negative aspects of self/world are focused on, and the positive overlooked. This worsens and maintains the depression. At the same time other symptoms occur:

 - **Physiological response** – biological symptoms of depression (poor sleep, appetite, etc.)

 - **Altered behaviour** – typically leads to **stopping** doing things in depression.

 The thinking errors and negative automatic thoughts (NATS) must be identified and challenged as part of the cognitive therapy approach. This can be done effectively in addition to medication/ electroconvulsive therapy, etc.

Table 4.1 Typical cognitive distortions (not an extensive list)[a]

Cognitive distortion	Definition
Black and white[b] **"All or nothing" thinking** Dichotomous/absolute thinking	The world/self and events are seen as extreme "black or white" interpretations with only two alternative possible beliefs being considered (e.g. *"Unless I do it perfectly, there's no point in trying"*)
Jumping to conclusions Overgeneralising Arbitrary inference	Drawing general conclusions from just one situation (e.g. *"I will never get better"*) just because one thing hasn't worked out as they would wish
Mental filter Minimising Magnification Selective abstraction	Negative or critical or threatening aspects of a situation are focused on and remembered at the expense of the positive, (e.g. *"Nothing ever goes right at work"*). The positive aspects of a situation or the person's actions are down-played (minimised) and negative aspects are focused on (magnification). Performance is underestimated while errors are overestimated
Mind-reading	The beliefs or future actions of others are assumed without any direct evidence for this, (e.g. *"They didn't really enjoy talking with me"*). Evidence to counter this is not sought by the person
Personalisation	The person takes responsibility for events that are not their responsibility, or feels that the actions of others are directed at themselves, (e.g. *"Its my fault that they didn't have a good time"*)
"Should"/"ought"/"must" statements	Absolute statements are made (e.g. *"I should always try my best or it's not good enough"*). As a result, it is likely that while the person holds this view, they will **never** be able to be happy
Catastrophising/ negative predictions/ **fortune telling**	It is believed that the very worst outcome will definitely happen, (e.g. in the middle of a panic attack *"I'll die/collapse/faint, etc."*)
Discounting the positive	The very many positive things that the person has done in the week are discounted and forgotten, e.g. the very real achievements of getting dressed and washed in someone with severe depression are discounted because *"I should be able to do that anyway"*, etc

[a] Summarised from a variety of different sources.
[b] **Bold** text indicates more "user-friendly" terms that may be used more easily with patients than the other terms mentioned.

These changes may be conceptualised as part of a **cognitive formulation** (illustrated in Fig. 4.1).

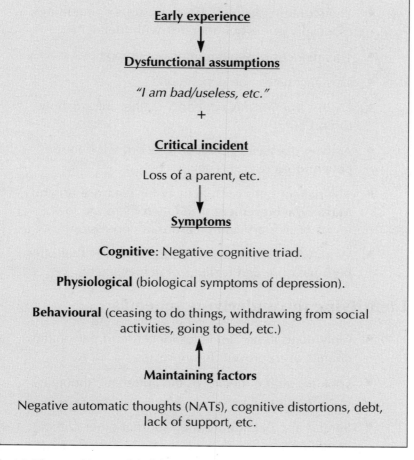

Fig 4.1　The cognitive model of depression.

Treatment is predominantly focused on challenging **unhelpful and inaccurate** underlying beliefs as described previously. In addition, behavioural approaches may also be used to reverse unhelpful behavioural changes. This can be an important part of treatment since:

- The underlying beliefs lead to altered behaviour.
- Depression leads to a loss of energy and anhedonia.
- Therefore the depressed patient stops doing things, especially going out, meeting with friends, etc.
- This reduces positive reinforcers (happiness) in life.
- This aggravates the depression.
- *"Is this true for this patient?"*. Gather information to find out.
- Activity diary can be used to record what the patient does over the next week.
- The patient rates each activity for **Pleasure** (P) and **Mastery/achievement** (M). Often there are low levels of mastery and pleasure in depression.
- Work with them to re-introduce activities that offer both pleasure and feelings of achievement.

Identifying the underlying schemas

- Only done if the aim is for longer term personality change or to prevent future relapse.
- Look for global themes in the automatic thoughts (e.g. *"I am bad"*).
- Similar approaches are used to treat other clinical conditions.

Downward arrow technique[4]

Try to identify the negative cascade of thoughts that occur, in order to identify the underlying schema; e.g. *"If it were the case that you had done the essay badly, what would be so bad about that?"*, which leads the patient to realise that *"I am useless"* – the underlying schema.

Cognitive Models of Anxiety

Three aspects to anxiety must be assessed:

- Cognitive.
- Physiological/bodily response.
- Behavioural.

Cognitive

Anxious preoccupation involves:

- Worrying – unhelpfully going over problems in a way that is unlikely to lead to their resolution.
- Negative predictions, catastrophising.
- Dwelling on: past regrets, present problems, future doubts.
- Hyper-vigilance causing anxious scanning of environment, restlessness and poor sleep.
- Possibly heightened consciousness of bodily sensations.

Bodily response

Physiological arousal causes physical sensations:

- Focus varies from person to person.
- Different patterns of stress reaction (headaches, eyestrain, abdominal pain, etc.) occur.
- Autonomic symptoms are very important.

Altered behaviour

Typically, the anxious person will start to **avoid** anxiety provoking situations (for example by avoiding entering large shops), or engage in a range of **safety behaviours** such as seeking reassurance from others or, in the case of panic, holding onto a physical support or sitting down in order to reduce their panic. According to the cognitive model, these avoidance and safety behaviours **must be altered** as part of the treatment plan because while they continue the person will never learn that the feared consequence (e.g. fainting) will not actually occur.

The Cognitive Model of Panic

Panic attacks occur when the patient becomes trapped in a *"vicious circle of panic"* (Fig. 4.2). The vicious circle is driven by the fearful thoughts that something terrible (and **catastrophic** such as dying, fainting or collapsing) will occur **imminently**. This increases arousal levels, thereby producing a range of autonomic and other sensations. These bodily sensations may then be misinterpreted by the patient as convincing evidence that the feared consequence will in fact occur. For example, in a patient who fears they are having a heart attack, the presence of a rapid heart and tenderness and tension in the superficial muscles of the chest wall may be convincing evidence to the patient that they are about to die. The presence of hyperventilation may produce sensations of chest pain and shortness of breath, blurred vision and dizziness. These may be misinterpreted as evidence that either the person is suffocating, or they may faint or suffer a stroke.

In each of these fearful circumstances, the behaviour of the patient flows logically from the beliefs they hold. The belief that they are about to faint may cause the patient to sit down or leave the room; the patient who fears they are suffocating may use their inhaler excessively, whereas those who fear they are having a heart attack may unsuccessfully use anti-anginal medication. If the symptoms continue, some patients may become so fearful that they dial for an ambulance and go to the Casualty department.

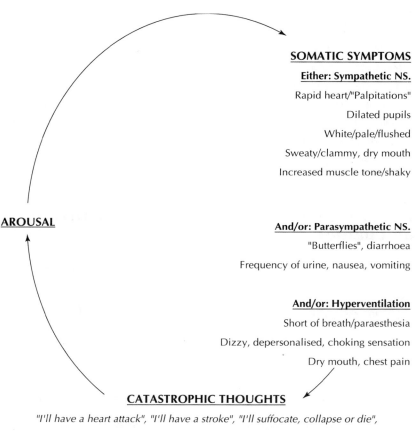

SOMATIC SYMPTOMS

Either: Sympathetic NS.

Rapid heart/"Palpitations"

Dilated pupils

White/pale/flushed

Sweaty/clammy, dry mouth

Increased muscle tone/shaky

AROUSAL

And/or: Parasympathetic NS.

"Butterflies", diarrhoea

Frequency of urine, nausea, vomiting

And/or: Hyperventilation

Short of breath/paraesthesia

Dizzy, depersonalised, choking sensation

Dry mouth, chest pain

CATASTROPHIC THOUGHTS

"I'll have a heart attack", "I'll have a stroke", "I'll suffocate, collapse or die",

"I'll make a fool of myself", "Everyone will be looking at me", etc.

BEHAVIOUR

Safety behaviour e.g. sit down, grab onto the shopping trolley, etc.

Avoidance: refuses to go to the supermarket, stay inside all the time, etc.

Fig. 4.2 Cognitive model of panic.[5]

The Cognitive Model of Generalised Anxiety

The cognitive model of generalised anxiety can similarly be explained by a vicious circle. Instead of the symptoms presenting with acute fear and panic, the fearful beliefs tend to focus on worry and negative predictions that things will go wrong (*"I'll never pass the exam"*, etc.). Cognitive distortions cause raised arousal levels which are accompanied by symptoms such as tiredness, irritability, and poor concentration and sleep. Behavioural changes such as avoidance tend to be more subtle than in panic; however, they may still act as a factor maintaining the anxiety. Again, the role of inaccurate and unhelpful thoughts is seen as central to causing and perpetuating the anxiety.

Cognitive behavioural treatment of anxiety and panic

1. **Gathering information** (diaries, etc.): to identify unrealistic catastrophic cognitions.

2. **Education**:

   - Effects of anxiety on the body.

   - The importance of tackling avoidance.

3. **Challenging catastrophic or unrealistic cognitions**:

   - Gather evidence, e.g. *"Will I really faint?"*.

   - Have they ever fainted? (They often haven't.)

   - *"Is it possible to faint as a result of panic?"* (It is not except in the rare case of blood phobia.)

   - *"Do you know what happens to someone's pulse when they faint?"* (It slows.)

   - *"What happens to your pulse when you feel like this?"* (It speeds up – check it next time they feel panicky.)

- Use a similar approach for whatever fears they have.

4. **Altering behaviour**: exposure and response prevention.

5. **Teaching skills to reduce causes of anxiety**:

  - Problem solving.

  - Relaxation.

  - Assertiveness.

  - Time management.

  - Distraction techniques.

  - Confidence building.

Cognitive Therapy of Phobias

Key figures: Isaac Marks (London).[6]

A phobia is defined as severe anxiety/fear focused on a particular thing leading to escape and avoidance behaviour:

- Exposure to the feared stimulus causes panic.

- Marked physiological arousal can be misinterpreted as evidence of impending doom.

- Catastrophic thoughts (*"I'll faint/collapse/die"*, etc.) occur.

Behaviour alters as a result, leading to:

- **Avoidance**: refusal to go anywhere near the feared place/situation (e.g. supermarkets).

- **Safety behaviour** (e.g. leaving the shop, sitting down, grabbing onto a wall, only going to the supermarket with a relative, etc.).

This can be very incapacitating.

Treatment of phobias

- Avoidance **maintains** the problem (they never come to realise that they **won't** die/collapse if they remain in the shop, etc.).

- They must **face up to the fear (exposure)**. By doing this their catastrophic fears will be shown to be inaccurate.

Treatment involves:

1. **Gathering information** (diaries, etc.).

2. **Education**:

   - Why they won't die.

   - Bodily arousal/effects of adrenaline.

   - Effects of hyperventilation (if present). Hyperventilate with them (a **behavioural test**) to show them the physiological effects that result.

3. **Challenging catastrophic cognitions**.

4. **Altering behaviour**:

   - Exposure (enter and stay in the shop).

   - Response prevention. (Don't run away/leave. Stick with the anxiety and it will improve. You **won't** die. The fear **will** improve/disappear.) This initially typically takes 20–60 minutes.

5. **Teaching skills to reduce causes of anxiety**.

Three styles of exposure

- Flooding.

- Systematic desensitisation.

- "Modelling" by therapist, (doctor/psychologist) or spouse who accompanies them and "models" being calm.

The best approach is a **graded (systematic) exposure**[7] (Fig. 4.3)

- Planned exposure with the patient.

- "Push" the person but not cause them to give up.

- Should aim for a cure in 3–4 weeks.

- Key is repeatedly facing up to the fear in a graded manner.

- Stick with the situation for at least 40 minutes or until the panic subsides.

- Exposure in treatment sessions, and also at home as "homework".

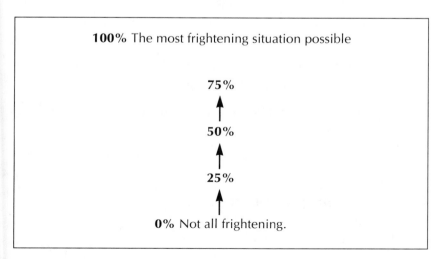

Fig. 4.3 Graded exposure (systematic desensitisation).

Obsessive–Compulsive Disorder (OCD)

Characteristics of obsessions and compulsions:

- They are seen as senseless and unpleasant.
- Recurrent, intrusive and excessive.
- The symptoms are unwanted and resisted by the person (they try to push them out of their mind).

Obsessions may be:

- Thoughts.
- Impulses.
- Images/pictures.

Compulsions are the motor equivalent of obsessions, e.g. cleaning, checking or other rituals.

A cognitive conceptualisation of OCD

- Focus is on something horrific to them (e.g. a mother may have thoughts of murdering her baby, a priest may have thoughts of blaspheming out loud, etc.).
- Each time the obsession is experienced, the person tries to push it out of their mind.
- **This avoidance perpetuates the problem** (they never learn that they will not actually blaspheme/murder the infant, etc.).

General principles of treatment[8]

- Gathering information (diaries, etc.).
- Education.

- Challenging catastrophic cognitions.

- Altering behaviour: **exposure and response prevention**. Help the person face up to their feared thoughts/images/impulses, etc.

Exposure and response prevention

- **Obsessions**: e.g. form the thought/image in their mind. Resist the temptation to immediately push the horrific thought out of mind.

- **Compulsions**: e.g. deliberately make the room dirty and leave it that way without cleaning it.

- Repeat this again and again.

Exposure to obsessional thoughts can include the following:

- The person records a graphic description of the thought/image on to a continuous loop of tape. They listen to this repeatedly for at least 30 minutes several times a day until the intensity and the extent of the obsessions diminish.

- Describe in detail the avoided thought/impulse/ image in the therapy sessions.

- Skills to reduce anxiety are taught, e.g. coping responses, distraction techniques, thought stopping.

- An elastic band "snapped" against the wrist can be a useful "springboard" for people to help them move their thoughts onto a different topic. Ulti- mately, the beliefs associated with the distressing experience must, however, be challenged.

These approaches can in each case be supplemented with specific medication aimed at either relieving depressive illness (antidepressants), or at aiding the effective treatment of the obsessive–compulsive disorder (e.g. selective serotonin re-uptake inhibitors).

Cognitive Model of Hypochondriasis

- The person has recurrent health anxiety and fears.

- "Normal" sensations are misinterpreted as reflecting illness.

- Catastrophic fears occur (*"I have cancer/heart disease/brain tumour/multiple sclerosis, etc."*).

- Preoccupation leads to increased fear and arousal which can then cause even more physical symptoms which are focused on and misinterpreted.

- They present repeatedly to doctors.

- They undergo multiple admissions or investigations.

- They are not reassured by this and continue to fear they have an illness.

- A vicious circle occurs, where they constantly look for evidence of illness by scanning their bodies for confirmatory evidence of the disease.

Treatment is similar to the treatment of anxiety alone, but also includes **re-interpreting the source of pain**, etc. (e.g. mental tension is causing tension in their muscles which is very painful. Behavioural tests such as pressing the muscles can help convince the patient that their muscles are tense and painful).

Post-Traumatic Stress Disorder (PTSD)

This is a mixed disorder, often presenting with various symptoms including a triad of:

1. Reliving the experience with recurrent intrusive images/flashbacks.

2. Overarousal, anxiety, panic, startle response, etc.

3. Avoidance of situations that invoke memories of the original stressor.

Affective symptoms are also common such as depression, guilt, etc.

Adopt a problem-orientated approach, treating each of the symptoms in turn:

- **Recurrent intrusive images**: Facing up to the feared thoughts/images; exposure and response prevention (form the avoided thought/image and keep it in mind). Use a similar approach to that in obsessional compulsive disorder (continuous loop tapes, etc.).

- **Anxiety**: cognitive treatments of anxiety; education, teach relaxation techniques, challenge catastrophic fears, etc.

- **Avoidance**: facing up to the fears; exposure and response prevention (systematic desensitisation).

- **Depression**: antidepressants/cognitive therapy of depression.

Problem Solving

Problem solving has been mentioned several times above. It is a very useful technique in cognitive therapy. The following model was described by Linda Gask, Jan Scott and Sally Standart.[9]

Is the problem realistic or unrealistic?

1. **Realistic**

    - **Resolvable**: offer problem solving.
    - **Unresolvable, unlikely to change**: offer coping resources and rally supports.

What are potential sources of outside help? How have they managed in the past? Use these strategies again.

2. **Unrealistic**: offer cognitive strategies.

Tablets can be offered in both cases.

Resolvable problems – problem solving

- It is a technique that can be learned.
- Practice leads to improvement.
- It works for any practical difficulties.
- Problems which seem enormous are often manageable.
- Need to approach it **one step at a time**.

According to Goldfried and Goldfried,[10] problem solving is a logical seven-step process:

1. Identify and **clearly define** the problem as precisely as possible.

2. **Brainstorm** multiple possible solutions. *"The more solutions you generate, the better"* (include ridiculous ideas as well initially).

3. **Assess** how effective and practical each suggestion is.

4. **Choose** one of the solutions.

5. **Plan out** the steps needed to carry it out.

6. **Do it!**

7. **Evaluate** the outcome; learn from any mistakes.

Key points

- Cognitive therapy appears to be an effective intervention for a growing range of psychiatric problems.

- Central to the cognitive model is the theory that beliefs affect emotional responses and behaviour. Challenging beliefs may be an effective intervention.

Cognitive models of different psychiatric disorders emphasise that inaccurate and unhelpful thoughts are central to maintaining the problem. Beliefs are challenged through education, hypothesis testing, generation of alternative explanations and behavioural experiments.

Suggested Further Reading

Blackburn, I M (1987). *Coping with Depression*. Edinburgh: Chambers.

Hawton K, Cowen P (eds) (1990). *Dilemmas and Difficulties in the Management of Psychiatric Patients*. Oxford: Oxford Medical Publications.

Hawton K, Cowen P (eds) (1992). *Practical Problems in Clinical Psychiatry*. Oxford: Oxford Medical Publications.

Hawton K, Salkovskis P M, Kirk J, Clark D M (eds) (1990). *Cognitive Behaviour Therapy for Psychiatric Problems: a Practical Guide*. Oxford: Oxford University Press.

References

[1] Kelly G A (1955). *The Psychology of Personal Constructs.* New York: Norton.

[2] Ellis A (1962). *Reason and Emotion in Psychotherapy.* Secaucus, NJ: Citadel.

[3] Beck A T, Rush A J, Shaw B F, Emery G (1979). *Cognitive Therapy of Depression.* New York: Guildford Press.

[4] Burns D D (1980). *Feeling Good: the New Mood Therapy.* New York: Signet.

[5] Clark D M (1990). Anxiety states. In *Cognitive Behaviour Therapy for Psychiatric Problems: a Practical Guide,* (eds) Hawton K, Salkovskis P M, Kirk J, Clark D M. Oxford: Oxford University Press.

[6] Marks I (1978). *Living with Fear; Understanding and Coping with Anxiety.* New York: McGraw Hill.

[7] Wolpe J (1958). *Psychotherapy by Reciprocal Inhibition.* Stanford: Stanford University Press.

[8] Salkovskis P M, Kirk J (1990). Obsessional disorders. In *Cognitive Behaviour Therapy for Psychiatric Problems: a Practical Guide* (eds) Hawton K, Salkovskis P M, Kirk J, Clark D M. Oxford: Oxford University Press.

[9] Gask L, Scott J, Standart S (1994). *Counselling Depression in Primary Care* (trainers' pack). London: Royal College of Psychiatrists.

[10] Goldfried M R, Goldfried A P (1975). Cognitive change methods. In *Helping People Change,* (eds) Kanfer F R, Goldstein A P. New York: Pergamon Press.

Chapter 5

The treatment of eating disorders

Chris Williams

The purpose of this chapter is to describe the treatment of the eating disorders (anorexia nervosa and bulimia nervosa). Many clinical text books outline the diagnosis, differential diagnosis and biochemical and physical changes that occur in anorexia nervosa and bulimia nervosa. These will not be specifically discussed here except where this affects treatment. Instead the focus will be on presenting information that may be used clinically with the patient to help them **understand** why they have developed an eating disorder, and to discuss ways in which effective treatment may be offered. This will particularly focus on the cognitive–behavioural treatment of both conditions.

Anorexia Nervosa (AN)

Key features:

- Very significant weight loss (at least 15% below expected for sex and height).

- First described by Gull[1] and Lasegue[2] independently in 1873.

- "Morbid fear of fatness";[3] "weight phobia";[4] "pursuit of thinness".[5]

- Loss of periods (amenorrhoea).

- May be associated with bulimia (AN–bulimic type).

Bulimia Nervosa (BN)

First described by Gerald Russell in 1979: *"An ominous variant of anorexia nervosa"*.[6]
Key features:

- Repeated binge eating.

- Craving.

- Very large quantities of food consumed.

- Regret/guilt as a result which leads to:

- Behaviour to reverse the potential weight gain due to the binge, including:

   (i)   Dieting that at times can be extreme (missing meals, self-starving, etc.).
   (ii) Self-induced vomiting.
   (iii) Abuse of laxatives.
   (iv) Abuse of other medications/dietary aids to lose weight (e.g. thyroxine, amphetamines, diuretics).
   (v)   Exercise may be undertaken with a view to losing calories rather than for fun.

Epidemiology

- This is useful to challenge the belief that they are the only person who thinks like this. They are not.

- 1 in 100 of 15–19 year old women has anorexia nervosa.[7]

- Rate of bulimia nervosa is not certain; but far more than the rate for anorexia nervosa.

- 25% of female university students have a significant binge-eating problem.

- Wide range of **normal** eating habits exists.

Cognitive Therapy

The essence of cognitive therapy is that what people think affects how they feel and act. People with eating disorders have characteristically extreme views concerning their weight and shape. These abnormal beliefs can be described as **overvalued ideas** (non-delusional beliefs, which if held to a minor degree can be said to be normal, yet instead are held with the greatest personal conviction and dominate the person's life to an unreasonable extent). Clinically, such patients could be described as showing *"Eating as a Way of Life"* which aptly describes the intense preoccupation with food.

The basis of treatment of both conditions includes:

1. **Assessment**.

2. **Education**: what eating disorders are, why they occur, what can be done to help.

3. **Interventions** (addressing the specific problem areas of the individual patient).

1. Assessment

The clinical assessment includes an eating history, physical examination and screening bloods.

Eating history

- How much do they weigh now?
- What is the expected weight of someone of their age, sex and height?
- Calculate the body mass index (BMI) (weight/height squared = 17.5 or less in anorexia).
- What is the most/least they have ever weighed?
- What is their "ideal" weight?
- Do they **feel** fat/overweight?
- Go through a "typical" day's eating.
- Is it difficult eating food (does it cause anxiety/distress)?
- Can they eat in company, or do they avoid this?

How do they control their weight?

- Low calorie intake/restricted food intake.
- Use of exercise to burn up calories rather than for fun.
- Abuse of laxatives, dietary aids or other tablets (amphetamines, diuretics, thyroxine, etc.). Faecal phenolphthalein levels can be carried out if covert laxative abuse is suspected.
- Self-induced vomiting (effects on teeth; Russell's sign – abraded knuckles caused by attempts to vomit, painless parotid gland enlargement).

Bingeing

- Can occur in anorexia **and** bulimia.

- What do they mean by a binge? By definition this must involve the eating of excessive food as part of a discrete meal. Some patients misuse this term to just mean a little over-eating.

Use of eating diaries

Eating diaries can be a useful way of gathering information. They have a number of different columns which record:

- What is eaten, when and where.

- Bingeing, vomiting, exercise or laxative use.

- Thoughts and feelings associated with that behaviour (*"I am fat"*, *"I hate myself"*, *"I have no control"*, etc.).

Diaries allow:

- A **clear record** to be kept. This can help challenge statements like *"nothing went well last week"*.

- **Patterns** can be identified so that times when the person is at risk of bingeing can be identified (just after returning from work, alone at night, etc.).

- Thoughts about shape and weight can be recorded at "key" times (just before being weighed, after a binge, etc.).

2. Education

Why do people develop eating disorders?

Anorexia typically affects:

- Women (female to male ratio is 15:1 for anorexia;[8] probably a similar figure is true for bulimia).

- Adolescence to thirties.

- Mainly the developed world. Very rare in the third world (although increasing amongst the middle and upper classes).

- **All** social classes (not just Social class I/II as thought previously).

Cultural pressure to slim

Western society stresses physical attractiveness through the media (advertisements, television, magazines, etc.). Higher than expected rates of anorexia occur in female models, athletes, professional dancers, private and boarding schools. The male equivalent may be athletes (e.g. marathon runners).

- Patients (and society) often see thinness as safe, attractive, controlled and good.

- This contrasts with fatness which is associated with being lazy ("slob"), uncontrolled, greedy, unfit and unattractive.

- These views are perpetuated by the media and culture in westernised countries at the present time (contrast this with different perceptions of what is attractive over the centuries (Hogarth's art), and in different places (e.g. Eskimos).

Other evidence of cultural focus on food

One important study examined the physical statistics of Playboy Centrefolds and Miss America Pageant Winners over a 20 year period:[9]

- **1959**: average Playmate weighed **91%** of the average population weight for women (actuarial figures).

- **1978**: fell to **83.5%** of the weight of the "average" women.

- The true weight of the average women under the age of 30 in the general population had actually **increased** over the same time period.

This mirrored a marked increase in the number of dietary articles in six women's magazines.
  Other studies have shown:

- Shop mannequins have become thinner over the years (some would be in hospital if they were alive!).

- Some supermodels seem almost (or actually) anorexic.

- Majority of women want to be slimmer.

- Majority of men want to be "beefier".

Other important areas to educate the patient about include the following.

Food as a symbol of love

- Learned in childhood.

- *"Eat up and be good"*.

- Sweets seen as a reward.

- Disobedience leads to the removal of food (punishment).

- Meals/food can become a focus of argument.

- Love/anger shown by eating/refusing to eat.

- Can "play out" anger at the meal table and express emotions that are not being expressed elsewhere.

Sometimes the only area of life in which the person feels they have any control is in the realm of eating.

- **"Comfort eating"** may involve emotions (e.g. anger, upset, guilt, anxiety) being expressed via eating.

Emotional and physical impact of the disorder

Emotional problems are often associated with eating disorders. In bulimia nervosa, the following problems are very common:

- Depression and guilt.

- Generalised anxiety.

- Panic attacks.

- Agoraphobia or social phobia.

- Poor concentration.

- Relationship problems at home and work.

- Low confidence and self-esteem.

In educating the person about the physical impact of starvation and/or bingeing:

- Talk in terms that the person can understand. If they are very thin, they need to know about the reality of the danger to their lives.

- Photographs can help make the point, e.g. of incisor damage as a result of self-induced vomiting.

- Describe the dangerous effects of vomiting (cardiac arrhythmias, low potassium), etc.

- Discuss areas that may be relevant to them: e.g. bulimia can cause problems such as spottiness, intermittent oedema, poor skin quality and irregular periods. This may add to motivation to change.

3. Interventions

Increase motivation to change (motivational interviewing)

To change, the motivation must come from themselves rather than others. A number of techniques can aid this.

- Generate a list of all the things:

  (i) That they have **stopped doing** because they are anorexic/bulimic.
  (ii) Things they would **like to do** if they didn't have this disorder.

- Producing lists examining the **advantages and disadvantages** of continuing how they are now may be helpful (e.g. people become frustrated by their behaviour, staying in all the time, losing their friends, etc.).

- Writing a "**back from the future**" **letter**. The patient is encouraged to write two letters. In the first one, they have to imagine that they are living in 10 years time, and they have overcome their problem; they are living a normal life, and doing the things they want to do. They must describe how good this is, and what advice they would give themselves to encourage them through the difficult times they are experiencing at the moment. In the second letter, they imagine that over the next 10 years there is no change – they have continued to be anorexic or bulimic over those 10 years. They must write the letter advising themselves how to avoid this situation occurring, and also describing how they predict they will feel in 10 years if things don't change at all.

Identify and challenge their thoughts about eating/shape and weight

Patients will have thoughts about themselves, their shape and weight that are inaccurate and unhelpful. They show the full range of cognitive distortions described in the cognitive therapy chapter (Chapter 4).

Identifying the thoughts

- From the clinical assessment (e.g. ask about attitudes to their current shape and weight, ideal weight, etc.).

- By noticing times when their mood changes very quickly (either worsening or improving).

- From eating or mood diaries.

- During weighing sessions.

- At times when they reveal their true shape, e.g. wear close fitting clothes, go swimming, look in the mirror.

- At interview, by asking questions such as *"if you put on two stones in weight, how would you feel?"*.

The overvalued ideas must be challenged and replaced with more objectively correct beliefs if there is to be a lasting recovery.

Challenging the thoughts

Information is emphasised which challenges their thinking, e.g. that:

- Laxatives have been shown to make little difference to food digestion, and their effects are short-lived and predominantly only due to changes in fluid balance.

- Self-induced vomiting is an ineffective form of weight reduction, and does not retrieve all the food that has been eaten.

What is the evidence for and against the beliefs that they have?

- Is it really true that they become objectively heavier as a result of eating one chocolate bar?

- When they feel fat and bloated, have they actually put on lots of weight?

- Does a weight rise of 0.5 kg really mean that they will put on many kilograms of extra weight?

Providing New Ways of Dealing with the Stressors in Life and Relationships

It is very important not to focus only on issues of food. This can often become a smokescreen which (although important) means that other areas like their anxiety, phobias, sexual and family issues, depression, assertiveness, problem solving and other relationship problems are overlooked. In many patients, these areas must be addressed or the person will not be able to show sustained improvement. Often the person's entire life and family relationships seem to revolve around their eating behaviour. Changing this focus can be very important.

Teach specific skills such as:

- Relaxation techniques.

- Assertiveness training (usually in a group).

- Social skills.

Also consider:

- **Family therapy**: Minuchin[10] used the term "**the psychosomatic family**", and describes pathological family interactions in some families with anorexic children including enmeshment, rigidity, and avoidance of conflict resolution. A superficial facade of family happiness may hide deep disillusionment, and the person's symptoms play a major role in family homeostasis, serving a role for both the person and their relatives. Occasionally, parents may only respond to their child when they are unwell, and unable to cope alone without close nurturing support. In support of this suggestion, Crisp *et al.*[11] found that the psychoneurotic state of the parents may worsen as the patient gained weight.

- It is often difficult to know whether this approach is fair. A "typical" mother and father do not exist.[12] It is both frustrating and demoralising for any parent to see their child harm themselves in this way, day after day, week after week, year after year. It seems to be the best clinical approach therefore not to be judgemental, but instead to assess in each case whether the relationship with the parents is helpful or unhelpful.

- Are others acting to **maintain** the problem?

- **High expressed emotion** has been shown to predict relapse in several psychiatric disorders.[13] Is there high expressed emotion in the family (critical comments, hostility and emotional over-involvement)?[14]

- Are they allowed the responsibility to make decisions and act in an adult and assertive way, or are they acting in an inappropriate child-like role?

Specific Points in the Treatment of Anorexia Nervosa

- Long-term 1:1 work is often needed.

- Focus is psychotherapeutic. Treat prominent depression.

- No specific drugs are useful for anorexia, although chlorpromazine is sometimes used to reduce tension/distress and (possibly) to increase appetite and body weight. Clinically, this does not seem to be very effective as a means of gaining weight.

- If weight falls below 40 kg, it is important that they receive a medical review. Sudden deaths can occur, particularly if the person is vomiting (low blood potassium as a result of vomiting causes the heart to stop). Referral to a specialist eating disorders service or requests for specialist advise would be indicated at that time.

Work to increase weight

Starvation causes anorexic pathology in "normal" people

Keyes *et al.*[15] in the "Minnesota Studies" examined American conscientious objectors who were systematically starved over a number of months. They developed a range of typically "anorexic" pathologies. They became obsessional and irritable, with a pre-occupation with food, bingeing, poor concentration, reduced libido, a reduction in outside interests and social withdrawal. They also inaccurately perceived themselves to be overweight. In the majority of these patients, these features disappeared with simple weight restoration.

Altered body perceptions

- Anorexics can accurately estimate the width of a "neutral" stimulus (block of wood or physical height), however systematically **overestimate** the true width of their own face, waist, chest and hips.[16] They overestimate the size of their own faces by over 50%. Although actually thinner, they **felt** themselves to be fatter than normal women.

- These misperceptions are corrected as weight is regained, and probably reflects a malfunction of the brain as the result of starvation.

- Putting on weight is an essential aspect of treatment, and one approach is to use **"food as medicine"** which must be **"prescribed"** three times a day.

- Liaison with a dietician is important so that an appropriate diet can slowly be re-introduced at a pace acceptable to both the patient and medical team, and also to help challenge inaccurate beliefs concerning food and its effects on the body.

To weigh or not to weigh?

- Some debate exists on this issue.[17] Does this unhelpfully focus on weight and ignore other issues? On balance, it seems essential to weigh anorexics as they receive treatment in order to measure improvement and detect relapse.

- Weighing should be carried out at a fixed time on defined days (body weight tends to fluctuate by several pounds from day to day and during the day).

- A "healthy weight range" is a more useful target to aim towards than one specific weight.

- Regular weighing can be a helpful final objective arbiter as to whether enough food is being eaten (*"the scales cannot lie"*).

- Thoughts and feelings when they saw their weight on the scales should be recorded and used as useful discussion material in treatment sessions.

Difficult Issues in Anorexia

End stage anorexia

- As weight drops below 30 kg, the person may experience faints, circulatory failure and sometimes cardiac arrhythmias due to low serum potassium. This requires:

  - Regular measurement of urea and electrolytes (for potassium).

  - Random measurement of blood sugar for hypoglycaemia.

  - Repeated measurement of blood pressure, pulse and temperature.

  - Regular weighing.

- Death tends to occur when the weight reaches around 25 kg. (caused by circulatory or respiratory failure, or infection).

- Under these circumstances, urgent medical assessment and consideration of nasogastric tube feeding under Section 3 of the Mental Health Act (1983)[18] should be considered. Legal precedents exist for use of the Mental Health Act to force admission to either a psychiatric or a medical ward for treatment (including forcible feeding such as by a nasogastric tube).

- Mortality rates depend on the selection of cases and the length of follow-up, leading to varying figures between 5%[19] and 18%.[20]

Rationale for using the Mental Health Act

- Death is possible with anorexia.
- Remission is possible even after many years (10 plus).
- The cognitive distortions and anorexic way of thinking may resolve with feeding.[15]

Main issues in coming to the decision are:

- Age and maturity of the person.
- Attitudes of relatives.
- Understanding of information/issues involved and capacity to consent.
- Dilemma of what to do next once they have put on weight – you can't tube feed forever.
- Any previous unsuccessful tube feeding.
- Removes control from the person.
- If the decision is made to allow the patient to stay as an out-patient in spite of extremely low weight, this can cause marked staff stress if the patient is obviously becoming very physically unwell (collapsing, very weak, very thin). Staff support and working as a team is important in this situation. Some centres now rarely, if ever, will feed someone forcibly.

Remember, **never give up hope**. Recent studies encourage the idea that recovery after even 10 years of severe anorexia is possible. Eckert *et al.*,[21] in a 10 year follow-up of 76 severely ill females with anorexia found that 18 (23.7%) had fully recovered. Overall, approximately half had a benign outcome, and only five patients had died (6.6%). A very poor outcome (death) was associated with an older age of onset (over 18), bingeing, vomiting, previous hospitalisation, and a previous very low weight at hospitalisation 10 years previously.

Out-patient or in-patient admission?

- Differing policies exist in different centres in the United Kingdom.

- Most anorexia patients are treated on an out-patient basis.

- Only admit if severe medical problems, or complex case and not improving (e.g. severe depression, suicidal, multi-impulsive problems, etc.).

- Have clear goals and a specific treatment plan.

Traditionally, there have been two main in-patient approaches:

1. **Behavioural regimes**:

   - Freedom to have visits/friends and watch television, etc., are contingent on eating and attaining specified behavioural targets (e.g. specific weight gains each week). Ethical aspects of this are debatable.

   - Can be successful, but many patients refuse to comply.

   - May well succeed in raising weight, but what happens after discharge?

- Does not teach patients the new skills that they will need to take charge of their own eating after discharge from hospital.

2. **Actively helping the patient to change their eating and attitudes about eating:**

   - Working **with** the patient. Long periods gaining trust/building up a relationship.

   - Exploring issues of control, sexuality, assertiveness and family and other relationships.

   - Sexual abuse appears to be a factor in some – particularly in bulimics.[22]

   - Outcome likely to be better with a trained team of specialised nurses working as part of a well planned Eating Disorders Team – the treatment of choice for moderate to severe forms of the illness particularly when chronic or very low weight.

The Multi-impulsive Patient with an Eating Disorder

This is defined as an eating disorder (especially bulimia) in the setting of a combination of other "impulsive" problems:

- Suicidal ideas and practice; self-cutting or chronic overdosing behaviour.

- Alcohol/drugs.

- Repetitive stealing or shop-lifting.

- Chaotic relationships.

- Can be very difficult to treat.

- Often occurs in the setting of sexual abuse.

- May have prominent depression and/or anxiety.

Treating the multi-impulsive patient

- Must have a clear treatment plan before you admit.

- Generate a "problem list" of the range of problem areas they have.

- Systematically instigate a treatment plan for those areas most likely to improve with reasonable input, e.g. treat depression, withdraw from alcohol, teach distraction and relaxation techniques, etc.

- Clear treatment plans exist for sexual abuse (e.g. Hobbs[23]).

Specific Points in the Treatment of Bulimia Nervosa

Identify the "vicious cycle of bulimia"[24] (Fig. 5.1)

The key point is that:

- The reversing behaviour (dieting, vomiting, laxatives, etc.) **maintains** the cycle.

- Therefore, break the cycle by re-establishing regular meals.

- Prescribe three regular "meals" a day.

- The size of the meals can be negotiated. They do not have to be very large at first.

- This may be supplemented by two or three snacks a day if wanted.

- Act to reduce craving (*"try it and see"*), therefore breaking the binge vomit cycle.

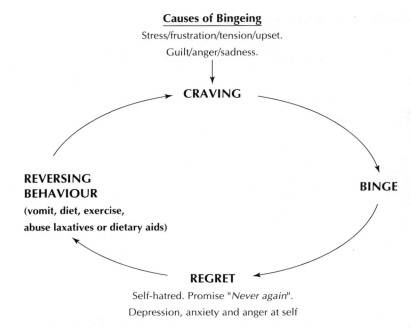

Fig. 5.1 The vicious cycle of bulimia.

- Patients fear an increase in weight: rarely happens (*"you will end up eating less"*).

To achieve this, other changes in behaviour are needed:

- Limit buying foods such as cake, bread, etc., that they are prone to binge on ("danger foods").

- Always plan the shopping and stick to the shopping list.

- Avoid impulse buying in the shop by carrying as little money as possible.

Avoiding the craving in the first place

- Use diaries to identify habits/patterns/difficult times when they are prone to binge (e.g. when alone/late evening, when upset, etc.).

- Avoid eating on "autopilot" (e.g. **eating without enjoyment** whilst watching television).

- Structure eating so that eating only occurs in the kitchen or dining room.

- **Limit** the supply of food available (through **selective shopping**, and by deciding how much food to cook).

- Choose foods that must be cooked, rather than biscuits, etc., that can be immediately eaten. They should only go for more when they have finished (*"re-train your stomach"*).

- Leave food and throw it away rather than bingeing on it. This can sometimes be **very** difficult.

- **Do not** leave supplies of food on the table (e.g. pots of honey/jam, etc.).

- Craving doesn't last forever and reduces after 20–60 minutes.

- Deal with the craving effectively early on in treatment by using **distraction techniques**.

- Patients may benefit from keeping busy at these times by making sure someone is there, telephoning friends, playing music, using relaxation skills, describing in detail an object in the room, etc. All these help the person cope with the craving until it subsides.

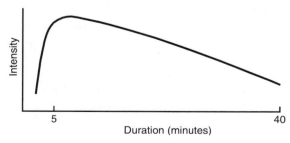

Fig. 5.2 The intensity of craving.

Other factors

- Treat prominent depression with antidepressants.

- If craving continues to be a problem, high dose fluoxetine (60 mg/day) may be helpful,[25] and it is likely that this is a class effect of selective serotonin re-uptake inhibitors.

- In the longer term, the treatment focus must move on to challenging and replacing unhelpful and inaccurate beliefs about shape, weight and eating. Without this it is unlikely that long-term benefits will be maintained.

- Relapse prevention work is an important aspect of treatment.

Key points

- Patients with anorexia and bulimia judge themselves in terms of their shape and weight.

- These beliefs are inaccurate and unhelpful. They cause emotional distress and alter behaviour in ways that add to the patient's difficulties.

- Management involves a full assessment of the cognitive, physical and social aspects of the presentation.

- Treatment is focused on both normalising eating behaviour, and also challenging unhelpful beliefs.

- It is important to address issues other than the eating problem alone. Issues surrounding control, relationships and coping strategies may all be important.

- In anorexia, the patient may need long-term input. Improvement is possible even after many years and the use of the Mental Health Act should be considered if death is a possibility.

References

[1] Gull W W (1873). Anorexia nervosa (apepsia hysterica). *British Medical Journal*, **2**, 527.

[2] Lasegue E C (1873). De l'anorexia hysterique. *Archives of General Medicine*, **21**, 385.

[3] Russell G F M (1970). Anorexia nervosa: its identity as an illness and its treatment. In *Modern Trends in Psychological Medicine*, vol. 2, (ed.) Price J H. London: Butterworths.

[4] Crisp A H (1967). Anorexia nervosa. *British Journal of Hospital Medicine*, **1**, 713.

[5] Bruch H (1973). *Eating Disorders*. New York: Basic Books.

[6] Russell G F M (1979). Bulimia nervosa: an ominous variant of anorexia nervosa. *Psychological Medicine*, **9**, 429–448.

[7] Crisp A H, Palmer R L, Kalney R S (1976). How common is anorexia nervosa? A prevalence study. *British Journal of Psychiatry*, **128**, 549–554.

[8] Crisp A H, Toms D A (1972). Primary anorexia nervosa or weight phobia in the male: a report on 13 cases. *British Medical Journal*, **I**, 334–338.

[9] Garner D M, Garfinkel P E (1980). Socio-cultural factors in the development of anorexia nervosa. *Psychological Medicine*, **10**(4), 647–656.

[10] Minuchin S (1974). *Families and Family Therapy*. Cambridge, MA: Harvard University Press.

[11] Crisp A H, Harding B, McGuinness B (1974). Anorexia nervosa, Psycho-neurotic characteristics of patients: relationship to prognosis. A quantitative study. *Journal of Psychosomatic Research*, **18**, 167–173.

[12] Crisp A H, Hsu L K G, Harding B, Hartshorn J (1980). Clinical features of anorexia nervosa: a study of a consecutive series of 102 female patients. *Journal of Psychosomatic Research*, **24**, 179–191.

[13] Kavanaugh D J (1992). Recent developments in expressed emotion and schizophrenia. *British Journal of Psychiatry*, **160**, 601–620.

[14] Vaughan C E, Leff J P (1976). The influence of family and social factors as the course of psychiatric illness. *British Journal of Psychiatry*, **129**, 125–137.

[15] Keyes A, Brozec J, Henschel A, *et al.* (1950). *The Biology of Human Starvation*, vols 1 and 2. University of Minnesota Press: Minneapolis.

[16] Slade P D, Russell G F M (1973). Awareness of body dimensions in anorexia nervosa: cross-sectional and longitudinal studies. *Psychological Medicine*, **3**, 188–199.

[17]   Touyz S W, Lennerts W, Freeman R J, Beumont P J V (1990). To weigh or not to weigh? *British Journal of Psychiatry*, **157**, 752–754.

[18]   The Mental Health Act (1983). London: Royal College of Psychiatrists.

[19]   Hsu L K G (1980). Outcome of anorexia nervosa: A review of the literature (1954–1978). *Archives of General Psychiatry*, **37**, 1041–1046.

[20]   Theander, S (1985). Outcome and Prognosis in anorexia nervosa and bulimia: some results of previous investigations, compared with those of a Swedish long-term study. *Journal of Psychiatric Research*, **19**, 493–508.

[21]   Eckert E D, Halmi K A, Marchi P, Grove W, Crosby R (1995). Ten year follow-up of anorexia nervosa: clinical course and outcome. *Psychological Medicine*, **25**, 143–156.

[22]   Waller G (1991). Sexual abuse as a factor in Eating disorders. *British Journal of Psychiatry*, **159**, 664–671.

[23]   Hobbs M (1990). Childhood sexual abuse: how can women be helped to overcome its long-term effects? In *Dilemmas and Difficulties in the Management of Psychiatric Patients*, (eds) Hawton, K, Cowen, P. Oxford: Oxford University Press.

[24]   Fairburn C, Cooper P (1990). Eating disorders. In *Cognitive Behaviour Therapy for Psychiatric Problems: a practical guide*, (eds) Hawton K, Salkovskis P M, Kirk J, Clark D M. Oxford: Oxford University Press.

[25]   Fichter M M, Leibl K, Rief W, Brunner E, Schmidt-Auberger S, Engle R R (1991). Fluoxetine versus placebo: a double blind study with bulimic inpatients undergoing intensive psychotherapy. *Pharmacopsychiatry*, **24**, 1–7.

Chapter 6

Difficult issues in liaison psychiatry

Peter Trigwell

Some areas of psychiatry are becoming increasingly high profile, with a consequent increase in the likelihood of questions being set on these areas in the exam. Liaison psychiatry is a particularly good example. It can be defined as "that area of psychiatry which is concerned with the diagnosis, treatment, study and prevention of psychiatric morbidity in the physically ill, of somatoform and factitious disorders, and of psychological factors affecting physical conditions".[1] A recent joint report by the Royal College of Psychiatrists and the Royal College of Physicians (*The psychological care of medical patients: recognition of need and service provision*) has helped to raise the profile of this sub-speciality, and developments are being made in the clinical setting.

Within the scope of liaison psychiatry there are some particularly difficult concepts (such as illness behaviour and somatisation) and complicated, ill-understood conditions (such as chronic fatigue syndrome). Many candidates will not have been fortunate enough to have worked in a liaison psychiatry training post. Such concepts and conditions will, therefore, be rather unfamiliar to them.

This chapter illustrates certain issues which are central to liaison psychiatry, by covering two important topics:

1. Illness behaviour and related concepts (including somatisation).

2. Chronic fatigue syndrome.

Illness Behaviour and Related Concepts

Terms

- Disease and illness.

- Illness behaviour.[2]

- The sick role.[3]

- Abnormal illness behaviour.[4]

- Somatisation.[5]

Disease and illness

- **Disease** is taken as referring to a disorder due to **organic pathology**.

- **Illness** is the **state experienced** by a person who perceives him or herself as suffering from ill-health.

Individuals vary enormously in how they respond to symptoms when ill. Some will make light of symptoms, shrug them off and avoid seeking medical care. They will continue to work as normally as possible, sometimes despite serious disease. Others will respond to the slightest evidence of ill-health by taking to their bed with a magazine and a bottle of Lucozade, and quickly seeking whatever medical help is available.

Illness behaviour

The concept of **illness behaviour** was first formally defined by **David Mechanic in 1961** as "the ways in which given symptoms may be differentially perceived, evaluated, and acted (or not acted) upon by different kinds of persons."[2]

Illness behaviour is a very important concept in medicine. It can be important in, and have an effect upon:

- Aetiology.

- Presentation (or not) to medical services.

- Diagnosis.

- Treatment.

- Prognosis.

Specific groups have been shown to differ with respect to their style of behaviour when ill:

- **Social class differences** were shown by **Koos in 1954.**[6] People of higher social class more often reported themselves ill than those of a lower class, and were also more likely to seek treatment when afflicted. This was despite the fact that lower social class people had more symptoms.

- **Cultural differences** also exist, shown by **Saunders in 1954**[7] when comparing Spanish and English speaking populations in south-western USA. "Anglos" preferred hospitalisation and modern medical science, the Spanish speakers tending to rely more upon folk remedies and family care.

Mechanic's 10 determinants of illness behaviour[8]

- Visibility, recognisability or **perceptual salience of signs and symptoms**.
- Extent to which symptoms are **seen as serious**.
- Extent to which symptoms **disrupt** family, work and other social activities.
- **Frequency** of appearance of signs or symptoms, their persistence or frequency of recurrence.
- **Tolerance threshold** of those exposed to signs and symptoms.
- **Available information, knowledge and cultural understandings** of those exposed.
- **Basic needs** that lead to denial.
- **Needs competing with illness responses**.
- **Competing interpretations** that can be assigned to recognised symptoms.
- **Availability of treatment** resources, physical proximity, plus costs of time, money, effort and **stigma**.

How people behave when perceiving themselves as ill has important implications for public health, estimating needs for medical care and addressing purchaser/provider issues. It is likely to be seen as increasingly important over coming years, therefore, but is also important for our general understanding of health and illness.

The sick role

The sick role is a concept developed by **Parsons in 1951**.[3] This is the special role in society occupied by a person who has declared him/herself as ill, and whose illness has been legitimised or "sanctioned" by a doctor (or cultural equivalent), or by relatives or friends.

Taking on the "sick role" involves **two main obligations**:

1. The person must **want to get well** as soon as possible.

2. They should **seek professional medical advice** and co-operate with the doctor.

And **two main privileges**:

1. The person is allowed (and perhaps expected) to **shed some normal responsibilities** and activities.

2. They are regarded as being **in need of care** and unable to get better by his/her own will.

In some situations there may be doubt as to whether the person actually has a "disease" (i.e. with recognisable organic pathology) to explain the symptoms of their "illness". The situation may then best be understood in terms of "abnormal illness behaviour" and "somatisation".

Abnormal illness behaviour

Abnormal illness behaviour is a concept developed by **Pilowsky in the 1960s**, drawing upon the aforementioned concepts of illness behaviour and the sick role. In essence, it refers to "inappropriately perceiving, evaluating and acting (or not acting) in relation to one's health".

Inherent within this is the conclusion by the doctor that the patient does not have appropriate objective pathology to entitle them to be placed in the type of sick role they are expecting, for the reasons for which they claim it.

Abnormal illness behaviour usually differs from normal in terms of quantity rather than quality, and attitudes are usually abnormal due to the fixity with which they are held rather than their content. This is an important area for research, and **Pilowsky** has developed the **Illness Behaviour Questionnaire** as a way of evaluating abnormal attitudes to illness.[9] Despite its widespread use, doubts remain about the validity of this measure.[10]

Somatisation

The concept of abnormal illness behaviour is very closely related to that of **somatisation**:

- First defined by Lipowski as "a *tendency to experience and communicate somatic distress and symptoms unaccounted for by pathological findings, to attribute them to physical illness, and to seek medical help for them*".[11]

- In its broadest sense refers to "*the expression of personal and social distress in an idiom of bodily complaints and medical help-seeking*".[5]

There is also a degree of overlap between somatisation and other, "older" concepts such as hysteria and hypochondriasis:

- Liaison psychiatrists tend to use the concept of somatisation as an **umbrella term**, with other concepts such as hysteria fitting within it. In other words, **somatisation** describes a **process or type of behaviour** (presenting/communicating psychological distress in the form of physical symptoms/complaints).

- This is distinct from **somatization disorder** (sometimes referred to as Briquet's syndrome) which is a specific disorder defined as "a history of many physical complaints or belief that one is sickly, beginning before the age of 30 and persisting for many years". The patient must have at least 13 physical symptoms from a list of 35, and there must be no pathophysiological mechanism to account for any of the symptoms being considered as supporting the diagnosis.[12]

- The following text addresses the broader concept of **somatisation**, not the specific syndrome known as somatisation disorder.

Note. The question of whether or not patients are "conscious" of producing physical symptoms without organic pathology is a clinical and ethical minefield. The doctor can never really know. A pragmatic approach should be taken in assessing and managing cases of somatisation.

Assessment and "diagnosis" of somatisation

As was always taught regarding hysteria, the "diagnosis" of somatisation should not simply be one of exclusion. After ruling out any organic pathology to explain the patient's symptoms, **certain features may make somatisation more likely as the explanation of the presentation**.

(a) Symptom characteristics

- **Quantity**: may be many different symptoms present, as in DSM-IV criteria for Briquet's syndrome.[12]

- **Consistency**: may be shifting between different symptoms, without the consistency expected in a case of disease due to organic pathology.

- **Quality**: may be highly emotionally laden and affectively charged descriptions of the pain or other symptoms.

- **Plausibility**: consider both the degree to which symptoms **cannot be fitted to a physical pathology** and the degree to which they **can be fitted to a psychological one**.

(b) Illness behaviours

- **Consulting behaviour**: in the individual consultation; in relation to medicine in general (e.g. multiple consultations/eagerness to seek medical help/possibly mixed hostility and dependence).

- **Social behaviour**: in the family; in the wider social role (e.g. "invalidity").

(c) Illness attitudes

- **Patient's ideas about**: the meaning of symptoms; the need for treatment; the importance of diagnosis; what doctors are like; the value of treatments.

Aetiology of somatisation

One must consider:

(a) Early factors in the history (vulnerability)

- Parents with chronic illness (i.e. learnt behaviour in childhood).

- Physical illness in early childhood (with benefits of the sick role/attention).

- Somatic vocabulary (more prominent in certain cultures, such as Nigeria and China).

- Alexithymia (lack of emotional vocabulary).

- Intellectual impairment affecting vocabulary/ expression of distress.

- Childhood neglect/regime of sympathy and attention for physical illness but not for emotional distress. The person would tend to communicate distress, or seek help/attention, by way of **physical complaints (symptoms) rather than emotional ones**.

(b) Later factors in the history (provocation)

- Stressors often have specific meaning for the patient; the stressor precipitating somatisation often has illness content, e.g. bereavement due to cancer or heart disease.

- May not be able to deal with the **distress** in normal way, so it presents as physical symptoms.

(c) Features of the illness

- Somatisation as a form of conflict resolution; the patient's illness and consequent invalidity/ dependence on others may be serving the purpose of keeping a relationship or family together. The sick role may enable avoidance of a distressing situation, perhaps at work. (Note – akin to concept of "primary gain").

(d) Sustaining factors

- Changed role.

- Changed relationships.

- Reduced social responsibility, etc.

Management of somatisation

Somatisation is common. The vast majority of such patients will present to general practitioners, physicians and surgeons rather than psychiatrists. One study found that 20% of patients who presented to their general practitioners with new episodes of illness had somatic complaints but without physical disease to account for their symptons.[13] Similarly, a recent British survey indicated that 20% of patients seen by neurologists do not have organic pathology to explain their symptoms despite appropriate – and often exhaustive – investigations.[14] In both studies, although some of these patients had some pathology it was not adequate to explain their symptoms and the ensuing disability.

There is a need to educate the doctors who see these patients, in order to facilitate both early recognition and appropriate treatment of this complex and potentially very costly problem. Also, the doctor's understanding of the problem and how he or she deals with it, discusses it with the patient and (if applicable) sets up psychiatric referral is crucial.

Ideally the initial treatment approach will be to:

- Elicit symptoms.

- Find the meaning of them to the patient.

- Carry out a physical examination and appropriate investigations.

- Give a clear diagnostic statement, i.e. what is **not** occurring and what **is** occurring.

- Explain pathophysiology of the symptoms.

- State and discuss the need for treatment.

Somatisation can be split into **acute** (weeks) **sub-acute** (up to 6 months) and **chronic** in duration. **With early and appropriate intervention the prognosis can be good**, avoiding a long period of illness with significant costs to the patient, their family and the health services.

Referral to psychiatric services is necessary for severe, chronic problems. Where a Liaison Psychiatry Service is available, a substantial proportion of referrals (30% according to Thomas[15]) will satisfy criteria for somatisation.

Management by the psychiatrist

- It is essential to **engage the patient** (may be very reluctant, or frustrated and hostile).

- **Acknowledge the failure** of traditional medical services to help them.

- **Acknowledge the reality** of their illness and symptoms.
- **Introduce the idea of a new approach** to assessment, symptom relief and improving quality of life (**not** concentrating on getting a diagnosis).
- The patient may remain very sceptical of a psychological approach to their problems. It may help to agree to a **limited period contract**, e.g. 3 months, during which time the patient will try the new approach. If the problem has not improved at all be the end of that time the patient may return to a physical approach. This technique avoids demanding that the patient gives up their illness beliefs immediately. It can be useful when trying to engage them in treatment.
- **Acknowledge concerns** about stigma and labelling.

Use **cognitive techniques**, spending time addressing and discussing attitudes to illness, medical care, etc. **The evidence the patient uses to support their beliefs is examined, along with possible alternative explanations**. Specific tasks can be used to test out alternatives (further details in Salkovskis[16]).

A **broadly behavioural approach** is used concomitantly with:

- Graded activities (gradually increasing, in a planned way).
- Changing social role (reducing invalidity).
- Reducing inappropriate consulting and consequent investigations.
- Reducing prescription of unnecessary medication.

It is also very important to **identify and address any issues/problems in the person's roles and relationships** which may be contributing to their distress or maintaining the somatisation:

- Are they in some sort of dilemma or conflict situation?

- Are the consequences of that situation being avoided or improved by the fact that they are ill and in the "sick role"?

- Is their illness preventing a worsening of their situation?

- Could it be seen as a way of keeping an otherwise failing relationship together?

Treatment is unlikely to be very successful without adequately identifying and addressing any such problem areas.

Treatment will usually be on an out-patient basis. In some cases, however, the degree of invalidity, or a difficult situation or relationship at home, **may warrant admission**. The (liaison) psychiatrist should be in charge of the patient's care. It can be extremely helpful to enlist the help of a **physiotherapist**. This is particularly the case if the presenting symptoms are weakness, paralysis or pain causing reduced activity, with consequent physical problems (muscle wasting, contractures, etc).

Note. In chronic somatisation, even if we accept that the process causing the symptoms is unconscious, it may seem impossible for the patient to "give up" their symptoms and move on without losing their dignity. A physical treatment, like physiotherapy, can provide them with an **"acceptable" reason for getting better**, as they may still not be able to openly accept the psychological nature of the cause of their symptoms.

Goldberg has also advocated **re-attribution of bodily symptoms**;[17] the three stages of this are covered largely in the approach suggested above, namely:

- **Feeling understood**.

- **Changing the agenda** (away from physical complaints).

- **Making the link** (between bodily symptoms and emotional disorder).

Speckens *et al.*[18] carried out a randomised controlled trial of cognitive behavioural therapy in patients with unexplained physical symptoms, and found that it was a "feasible and effective treatment" in these patients.

Medication

There may also be a place for medication. In many patients with functional somatic symptoms (somatisation) evidence for an affective disorder can be found. Depending upon the nature of these symptoms it may be helpful to consider:

- **Tricyclic antidepressants**: for depressive symptoms, anxiety, panic and pain (some of these drugs are now licensed as analgesics and are particularly helpful in atypical or chronic pain).

- **SSRIs**: again, for depressive symptoms, anxiety, etc., especially if tricyclics are contraindicated by patients physical condition (**remember that somatising and having an organic disease are not mutually exclusive**!)

- **MAOIs**: especially in an "atypical" depressive picture.

- **Benzodiazepines**: should largely be avoided due to possibility of dependence.

- **Beta-blockers**: possibly helpful in anxiety states involving marked autonomic symptoms with lack of psychic anxiety.

Overall approach

The overall approach should be **eclectic and flexible**, with the emphasis on the psychological techniques outlined above. It is important to remember that "**chronic somatisers**" **are particularly demanding to treat**. A recent review paper commented that the aim may have to be "**damage limitation**" (control of medical care, reducing disability, help for relatives) rather than cure.[19]

One strategy for damage limitation in **severe cases** relates to the response to repeated presentations at hospital, with consequent investigations which are costly and carry risks to the patient. The situation may be brought more under control by a **clear statement** at the beginning of the patient's notes about what the problem is. Essential investigations should be carried out but (if they are negative) the patient should then be transferred to the care of the **same named consultant on every occasion**. This may be a physician who knows the patient and the situation well, or the liaison psychiatrist. The aim is to avoid risks and costs to the patient and attempt, repeatedly if necessary, to engage them in the management approach to their problem which is described above.

Chronic Fatigue Syndrome

The symptom of chronic fatigue is a feature of many disorders. Sometimes, however, there is no obvious disorder to explain the fatigue in patients who have this as their main complaint. The status of this so-called **chronic fatigue syndrome (CFS)** is a continuing area of controversy.

Two forms exist:

- **Epidemic form**: has been termed epidemic neuromyasthenia, Royal Free Disease, Icelandic disease and epidemic myalgic encephalomyelitis.

- **Sporadic form**: has been termed myalgic encephalomyelitis (ME) and post-viral fatigue syndrome (PVFS).

Historical background

There are some problems in looking at historical accounts, as pre-1900 physicians had even more difficulty than their modern day counterparts in distinguishing "psychogenic" from "neurogenic" weakness. Thus, patients referred to as "exhausted" could have been suffering subjective fatigue or objective paresis of the muscles.[20]

The history of CFS would appear to be long, despite such modern names for it as "the malaise of the 1980s" and "yuppie 'flu". Idiopathic chronic fatigue as the primary complaint was rarely reported before the late 19th century, but the condition appears to have existed before this under several different names:

- **Eberhard Gmelin** described such patients **in 1793**.

- **Weir Mitchell** wrote about such patients in the **1800s**.

- There was a particular rise of accounts in the last 30 years of the 19th century.

- It is possible that CFS is basically the same condition as the previously common diagnosis **neurasthenia** (named by **John Brown in 1780** and popularised by **George Beard**[21, 22] between **1869 and 1880**).

Aetiology of chronic fatigue syndrome

Evidence has been put forward to attempt to support various aetiologies:

- Specific viral infections (notably Epstein–Barr virus).

- Abnormal immune function, including the persistence of viral immune response.

- Abnormalities of the hypothalamic–pituitary–adrenal axis.

- Electrolyte abnormalities.

- Muscle abnormalities (including findings on single fibre EMG and abnormal mitochondria).

- Masked depression.

Despite this, the findings have generally not been replicated and the aetiology of the condition remains unclear. The term "chronic fatigue syndrome" was suggested as a replacement for earlier terms (such as myalgic encephalomyelitis, ME) as it is descriptive and free from unproven aetiological implications.[23] It is almost certainly multifactorial, and those who see it as a psychiatric problem often consider it to be a form of somatisation (see above section). In support of this, the rate of DSM-III somatisation disorder in patients with CFS is 10–15%, which is at least three times as high as in other medical populations and 10–20 times as high as in community samples.[24]

Thus, concepts useful in understanding the onset of CFS **may** include:

- History of early physical illness (in patient or family).
- Early regime of attention for physical illness but not for emotional distress.
- Somatic vocabulary/alexithymia.
- Relationship and role difficulties.
- Dilemma/conflict resolution.
- Primary and secondary gain.
- Illness attribution and stigma.
- Meaning of stressors.

(See section on somatisation, above, for more details.)

Diagnosis/classification in chronic fatigue syndrome

In view of the frequency of this condition, its costs and the increasing amount of research, it is essential to be able to compare studies in a meaningful way. This has been very difficult due to the wide range of disciplines involved in the research, each with a different approach and vocabulary. Sharpe,[25] has listed the different clinical syndromes which all appear to relate to the same group of patients:

- Epidemic neuromyasthenia.

- Idiopathic chronic fatigue and myalgia syndrome.

- Benign myalgic encephalomyelitis.

- Chronic infectious mononucleosis.

- Royal Free disease.

- Post-viral fatigue syndrome.

- Fibrositis–fibromyalgia.

- Chronic fatigue syndrome.

- (Neurasthenia could be added to the list.)

The need for a common diagnosis/classification system for this disorder led to:

- **Centre for Disease Control (CDC) criteria, 1988:**[23] these criteria were too complex and narrow.

- **Lloyd's criteria, 1988:**[26] concentrated on fatigue following physical but not mental effort.

- **The Oxford criteria, 1990:**[27] followed a consensus meeting of 21 workers in the field from varied backgrounds. This produced useful criteria which summarise what most clinicians working in this area mean by "CFS".

The Oxford criteria for a diagnosis of chronic fatigue syndrome:

- A syndrome characterised by **fatigue as the principal symptom**.

- A syndrome of **definite onset** that is not life long.

- The fatigue is **severe, disabling, and affects physical and mental functioning**.

- The symptom of fatigue should have been present for a **minimum of 6 months** during which it was present **for more than 50% of the time**.

- Other symptoms may be present, particularly myalgia, mood and sleep disturbance.

- **Certain patients should be excluded from the definition**. They include:

  (i) Patients with established medical conditions known to produce chronic fatigue (e.g. severe anaemia). Such patients should be excluded whether the medical condition is diagnosed at presentation or only subsequently. All patients should have a history and physical examination performed by a competent physician.

  (ii) Patients with a current diagnosis of schizophrenia, manic depressive illness, substance abuse, eating disorder or proven organic brain disease. Other psychiatric disorders (including depressive illness, anxiety disorders, and hyperventilation syndrome) are not necessarily reasons for exclusion.

Presentation of chronic fatigue syndrome

In line with the above criteria, most patients present with a history of:

- At least several months of fatigue, which is affecting daily functioning.

- It is both physical and mental fatigue.

- They have occasional good days when they can be active but, if they exert themselves, will then suffer extreme fatigue for several days or more (this is a pattern characteristic of patients with CFS).

- Marked myalgia.

- Some depression/anxiety symptoms.

They present mainly to general practitioners, but are sometimes referred on to a hospital (usually the infectious diseases or neurology clinic) for further investigation if symptoms persist. This is to rule out any organic pathology which could explain their symptoms. Multiple physical investigations are likely to be carried out, to exclude any such organic cause of the symptoms:

- Full blood count.

- Plasma viscosity.

- Urea and electrolytes.

- Liver function tests.

- Calcium estimation.

- Creatinine kinase.

- Random blood glucose.

- Thyroid function tests.

- Immunoglobulins.

- T-cell subsets.

- Anti-nuclear factor.

- Rheumatoid factor.

- Assays for: Epstein–Barr virus; Cytomegalovirus; *Toxoplasma gondii*; *Brucella*; Coxsackie virus.

- Plain chest radiograph.

In practice, the symptom profile outlined above with negative results from these tests will lead to a diagnosis of CFS.

Management of chronic fatigue syndrome

It is essential to take a **pragmatic approach** to managing this condition. Some of the principles of treating somatisation (outlined in the previous section) may be helpful. A useful model is to have **liaison psychiatry** input into the infectious diseases clinic, the patient being referred on to the psychiatrist after the medical assessment.

How the referral is suggested by the medics is very important. It can be done well if close liaison is maintained between teams. (Of the first 100 such patients at the Leeds Chronic Fatigue Clinic, only one refused referral to liaison psychiatry.)

1. **Engage the patient** (may be very reluctant, or frustrated and hostile):

   - **Acknowledge failure** of traditional medical service to understand CFS or help them.

   - **Acknowledge the reality** of illness and symptoms.

   - **Introduce the idea of a new approach** to assessment, symptom relief and improving quality of life.

   - Discuss importance of **psychological as well as physical aspects**.

- In practice, need to use a **biopsychosocial approach** (addressing physical, psychological and social factors).

- Discuss and acknowledge **effects of chronic illness** on psychological well-being (depression, self-esteem and anxiety), roles and functioning, relationships, etc.

It is important to bear in mind the fact that patients with chronic fatigue syndrome have **no identifiable organic pathology to explain their symptoms**. In acute illnesses, adoption of the sick role is temporary – often because the illness is treatable. In the case of chronic illness, however, broader issues of communication and identity are important for the patient's understanding of their illness and coping strategies. They have to continue to live with their illness indefinitely. According to Radley,[28] chronic illness is not adequately explained by the concept of the sick role, because "in addition to the role of patient, being chronically ill involves relationships with the healthy who express (both) compassion and abhorrence towards the sick". The negative ("abhorrence") component, in health professionals and others, may be increased if the patient lacks an identifiable organic pathology to justify their sick role. Perception of this by the patient would be likely to adversely affect their confidence in and, therefore, the efficacy of the health care they receive.

2. **Full psychiatric assessment**:

- To rule out any formal psychiatric disorder which has been missed and requires treatment.

- Any such disorder which is discovered can be addressed in the usual way.

3. **Education and graded activity**:

- **Avoid total inactivity**.

- Discuss **effects of prolonged inactivity**, with

significant muscle bulk being lost in 1 week, and further loss continuing with continued low levels of activity.

- Consequent weakness and muscle pain upon resuming activity, and "taking to bed" again as a result, leads to the setting up of a **vicious cycle**.
- **Increase activity** in a gradual, planned and **graded way**.
- **Avoid overactivity** on the occasional "good days" (which would be followed by prolonged worsening of fatigue).
- **Group work** can be useful, and **occupational therapist** input is invaluable.
- **Cognitive therapy approaches** are also important (see Chapter 4).

4. **Appropriate medication**:

- Some find traditional **analgesics** helpful for myalgia.
- **Antidepressants** (e.g. tricyclic antidepressants) are helpful in many cases, for several reasons:
  (i)   **analgesic** effects.
  (ii) **anxiolytic** (re. tension/myalgia).
  (iii) if **depressed**.
  (iv) to help **insomnia** (surprisingly frequent in CFS).
  (v)   possible beneficial effects on the **immune system**.

It is essential to **stress this rationale** for using these drugs, and that they are not generally being used primarily for their antidepressant action. Also explain to the patient:
  (i)   They are not addictive.
  (ii) It is important to persevere before stopping.
  (iii) Expected side effects.
  (iv) They are useful **as part of the overall attempt to move on** and improve the patient's situation.

Other approaches

- **Sharpe**[25] and **Butler**[29] have both advocated a similar approach, using cognitive and behavioural principles. A randomised controlled trial has been reported by Sharpe *et al.*,[30] which showed significantly better improvement in functioning in the group treated with cognitive behaviour therapy than a group receiving traditional medical care.

- Wholly biological treatments have been advocated, but often later rejected. In 1990, two contradictory reports appeared in the same journal: an Australian group reported **good** results using intravenous IgG; the very next paper, however, was from an American group and reported that it was **not** of clinical benefit!

Reports abound in the **media** regarding theories of causation and suggested "cures" for this condition, including:

- Removal of dental fillings.

- Various exclusion diets.

- "Anti-allergy" injections.

- Herbal remedies.

- Acupuncture.

- Anti-fungal treatments.

There may indeed be a place for some elements of some of these approaches. Unfortunately, however, the remedies so far advertised have two main features in common; a **total lack of well-controlled trials of efficacy**, and a **high cost to the patient**. In the immediate future the most pressing requirement is for good, large, methodologically sound and well-controlled trials of the efficacy and effectiveness of treatment approaches.

The aetiology of chronic fatigue syndrome will hopefully become clearer in time, although the reluctance of some to accept the possible part played by psychological mechanisms does not help this advance. The name may change again, or new ones may appear to confuse the picture further, but effective treatment is what is needed more than anything for the benefit of a large number of seriously debilitated people and their families.

Prognosis in chronic fatigue syndrome

There are few data, and they are inconclusive:

- Sharpe,[31] found that attributing the cause to solely physical factors was a predictor of ongoing disability at 2-year follow up.

- Wilson,[32] in Australia showed disappointing results; most improved over time but only 6% were fully recovered after 3 years. (This is a group who are severe and chronic enough to justify tertiary referral, however.) Wilson also commented that, in CFS, "subjects who deal with distress by somatisation . . . and who discount the possible modulating role of psychosocial factors are more likely to have an unfavourable outcome".

Suggested Further Reading

- Bass C (1990). *Somatization: Physical Symptoms and Psychological Illness.* London: Blackwell Scientific Publications.
- Creed F, Mayou R, Hopkins A (1992). *Medical Symptoms Not Explained by Organic Disease.* London: Royal College of Psychiatrists and Royal College of Physicians.
- Dawson A M, Creed F H et al. (1995). *The Psychological Care of Medical Patients: Recognition of Need and Service Provision.* London: Royal College of Physicians and Royal College of Psychiatrists.
- House A, Mayou R, Mallinson C (1995). *Psychiatric Aspects of Physical Disease.* London: Royal College of Physicians and Royal College of Psychiatrists.

- Salkovskis P M (1990). Somatic problems. In *Cognitve Behaviour Therapy for Psychiatric Problems: a Practical Guide*, (eds) Hawton K, Salkovskis P M, Kirk J, Clark D M. Oxford: Oxford Medical Publications.

References

[1] Bass C M (1995). The role of Liaison Psychiatry. In Psychiatric Aspects of Physical Disease, (eds) House A, Mayou R, Mallinson C. London: Royal College of Physicians and Royal College of Psychiatrists.

[2] Mechanic D (1961). The concept of illness behaviour. *Journal of Chronic Diseases*, **15**, 189–194.

[3] Parsons T (1951). *The Social System*. New York: Free Press of Glencoe.

[4] Pilowsky I (1969). Abnormal illness behaviour. *British Journal of Medical Psychology*, **42**, 347–351.

[5] Kleinman A, Kleinman J (1985). Somatisation: the interconnections in Chinese society among culture, depressive experiences, and meaning of pain. In *Culture and Depression. Studies in the Anthropology and Cross Culture Psychiatry of Affect and Disorder*, (eds) Kleinman A, Good B. London and Berkeley: University of California Press, pp. 429–490.

[6] Koos E (1954). *The Health of Regionsville: What the People Thought and Did About It*. Columbia: University Press, New York.

[7] Saunders L (1954). *Cultural Differences and Medical Care*. New York: Russell Sage Foundation.

[8] Mechanic D (1977). Illness behaviour, social adaptation and the management of illness. *Journal of Nervous and Mental Disease*, **165**, 79–87.

[9] Pilowsky I, Spence N D (1983). *Manual for the Illness Behaviour Questionnaire (IBQ)*, 2nd edition. Adelaide, Australia: University of Adelaide.

[10] Trigwell P J, Hatcher S, Johnson M, Stanley P J, House A O (1995). "Abnormal" illness behaviour in chronic fatigue syndrome and multiple sclerosis. *British Medical Journal*, **311**: 15–18.

[11] Lipowski Z J (1988). Somatization: the concept and its clinical application. *American Journal of Psychiatry*, **145**, 1358–1368.

[12] American Psychiatric Association (1994). *Diagnostic and Statistical Manual of Mental Disorders*, 4th edition. Washington D.C.: American Psychiatric Association.

[13] Goldberg D P, Bridges K W (1988). Somatic presentations of psychiatric illness in primary care settings. *Journal of Psychosomatic Research*, **32**, 137–144.

[14] Mace C J, Trimble M R (1991). "Hysteria", "functional" or "psychogenic"? A survey of British neurologists preferences. *Journal of the Royal Society of Medicine*, **84**, 471–475.

[15] Thomas C J (1983). Referrals to a British liaison psychiatry service. *Health Trends*, **15**, 61–64.

[16] Salkovskis P M (1990). Somatic problems. In *Cognitive Behaviour Therapy for Psychiatric Problems: a Practical Guide*, (eds) Hawton K, Salkovskis P M, Kirk J, Clark D M. Oxford: Oxford Medical Publications.

[17] Goldberg D, Gask L, O'Dowd T (1989). The treatment of somatisation: teaching techniques of reattribution. *Journal of Psychosomatic Research*, **33**, 689–695.

[18] Speckens A E M, van Hemert A M, Spinhoven P, Hawton K, Bolk J H, Rooijmans G M (1995). Cognitive behavioural therapy for medically unexplained physical symptoms: a randomised controlled trial. *British Medical Journal*, **311**, 1328–1332.

[19] Sharpe M, Peveler R, Mayou R (1992). The psychological treatment of patients with functional somatic symptoms: a practical guide. *Journal of Psychosomatic Research*, **36** (6), 515–529.

[20] Shorter E (1993). Chronic fatigue in historical perspective. In *Chronic Fatigue Syndrome* (Ciba Foundation symposium **173**), (eds) Kleinman A, Strauss S E. Chichester: Wiley, pp. 6–22.

[21] Beard G (1869). Neurasthenia or nervous exhaustion. *Boston Medical and Surgical Journal*, **3**, 217–220.

[22] Beard G (1880). *A Practical Treatise on Nervous Exhaustion (Neurasthenia).* New York: William Wood.

[23] Holmes G P, Kaplan J E, Gantz N M *et al.* (1988). Chronic fatigue syndrome: a working case definition. *Annals of Internal Medicine*, **108**, 387–389.

[24] CIBA Foundation Symposium 173 (1993). *Chronic Fatigue Syndrome*, (eds) Kleinman A, Strauss S E. Chichester: Wiley.

[25] Sharpe M (1990). Chronic fatigue syndrome: can the psychiatrist help? In *Dilemmas and Difficulties in the Management of Psychiatric Patients*, (eds) Hawton K, Cowen P. Oxford: Oxford University Press.

[26] Lloyd A R, Wakefield A, Boughton C, Dwyer J (1988). What is myalgic encephalomyelitis? *Lancet*, **i**, 1286–1287.

[27] Sharpe M (1991). A report – chronic fatigue syndrome: guidelines for research. *Journal for the Royal Society of Medicine*, **84**, 118–121.

[28] Radley A (1994). *Making Sense of Illness.* London: Sage Publications.

[29] Butler S, Chalder T, Ron M, Wessely S (1991). Cognitive behaviour therapy in chronic fatigue syndrome. *Journal of Neurology, Neurosurgery and Psychiatry*, **54**, 153–158.

[30] Sharpe M, Hawton K, Simkin S, Surawy C, Hackman A, Klimes I, Peto T, Warrell D, Seagrott V (1996). Cognitive behaviour therapy for the chronic fatigue syndrome: a randomised controlled trial. *British Medical Journal*, **312**, 22–26.

[31] Sharpe M, Hawton K, Seagrott V, Pasvol G (1992). Follow up of patients presenting with fatigue to an infectious diseases clinic. *British Medical Journal*, **305**, 147–152.

[32] Wilson A, Hickie I, Lloyd A, Hadzi-Pavlovic D, Boughton C, Dwyer J, Wakefield D (1994). Longitudinal study of outcome of chronic fatigue syndrome. *British Medical Journal*, **308**, 756–759.

Chapter 7

Practical child psychiatry (within a child mental health team)

Barry Wright

Child psychiatry is one of the subjects which is listed as a *sub-speciality* for the purposes of the essay paper. It is an area which lends itself well to essay questions. Consequently it will appear on the paper with increasing frequency, particularly since two of the four questions will now always be set on sub-speciality subjects. This chapter is in three parts. First, the complex topic of Abuse in Childhood; secondly, an outline of Practical Treatments in Child Psychiatry; and finally, the particularly important topic of Family Therapy.

Treatment of Abuse in Childhood

Assessment and treatment

There are different types of abuse that may occur in childhood. These include:

- Emotional abuse and neglect[1] (see Thompson and Kaplan[2] for a recent review).

- Physical abuse.[3]

- Sexual abuse.[4]

- Munchausen by proxy.[5]

Abuse affects the child in different ways depending on many factors including the age, sex and temperament of the child; the type, extent and perpetrator(s) of the abuse; the response of those in the child's environment, and so on. Your essay will need to be adapted to suit the question (for example for the type of abuse specified).

Statistics are thought to underestimate the extent of the true situation:

- 4% of children under 12 each year are brought to attention of agencies (NSPCC, etc.).

- 0.4% of children under 18 are on a child protection register.

- 0.1% of children under 16 are in care.

Epidemiology

A discussion of the definitions (found in many textbooks) and epidemiology of abuse will be essential. Tailor this to the type of abuse. For example, physical abuse is more likely with:

- Lower socio-economic families.

- Poor social support.

- High family stress levels.

- Poor quality of parental relationship.

- Large family.

- Very young mothers.

- Boys are more at risk as children than adolescents, girls more at risk as adolescents.

Adolescents are more likely to be abused:

- If they live in families with step-parents.

- With authoritarian/over-punitive, or over-indulgent parenting.

You should use your reading to produce lists describing the risk factors for those who are at risk of other types of abuse, but many of the above factors are shared.

Effects of abuse

The effects are variable depending on the many factors (child, parental, family, environmental) mentioned above. In the essay, consider the specifics of the question carefully (e.g. type of abuse) and long-term and short-term effects. Consider the impact on the child:

- **Emotional** (e.g. post-traumatic stress disorder, psychosexual problems).

- **Physical** (e.g. brain damage, scarring).

- **Social** (e.g. rejection, social phobia, over-protective parenting).

For example, if asked about the short- to medium-term effects of sexual abuse, **Finkelhor**'s[6] model of dynamics suggests the following changes:

- Inappropriate sexualisation or regression.

- Betrayal of trust and associated loss (control, family, virginity, etc.).

- Stigma/guilt.

- Powerlessness.

Changes which have been described by other authors include low self-esteem, self-harm, fear, isolation, secrecy, confusion, anger (against oneself or the family as well as towards the perpetrator), poor concentration and learning problems. Psychiatric illnesses which have been associated with sexual abuse include post-traumatic stress disorder, anxiety, depression, eating disorders, enuresis/encopresis, phobias, recurrent nightmares and dissociative states. In the **child sexual abuse accommodation syndrome**[7] the child sees him/herself as responsible. There will also be dysfunctional relationships associated with abuse.

Factors that influence effects, prognosis and planning of treatment

1. **Child factors**:

   - Age, sex and developmental status.

   - Temperament. (The concept of **grooming** implies that some abusers select and prepare certain children they intend to abuse.)

   - Emotional resilience and other coping strategies.

   - Feelings about (response to) disclosure, investigation, and court procedures.

2. **Abuse factors**:

   - Type and circumstances of abuse.

   - Nature of abuse (penetration of the vagina or anus and the use of violence carry a worse prognosis).

   - Associated factors (e.g. threats, coercion, bribery).

3. **Parental factors**:

- Personality factors, poor parenting skills, negative attributional styles, mental state (e.g. maternal depression), drug dependence and being in a family with a step-parent are all felt to be relevant.

- Other factors include a past history of abusing children and certain types of criminality, as well as past experiences of being in care or being abused as a child oneself. There have been variable findings in studies looking at transgenerational influences.

- Response to disclosure.

4. **Family factors**:

- Family support.

- Levels of stress in family.

- Consequences of disclosure (disintegration, rejection, retaliation, persecution, believed or blamed).

5. **Environmental factors**:

- Levels of support for family/parents.

- Poor socio-economic circumstances.

- Involvement of agencies.

In deciding **treatment** options, it is pertinent to consider **whether changes are possible**. For example, can the parents make use of therapy? Parents physically abusing their children may have:

- Unrealistic expectations of child behaviour (e.g. *"She is a naughty baby, she cries at night"*).

- Poor problem-solving skills and parenting strategies.

- Poor anger management.

- Poor social skills.

Interventions

General principles after abuse has come to light[8]

- Child's safety is paramount.

- Notify social services promptly (confidentiality waived). An **at-risk register** enquiry should be made.

- There are issues around confrontation. If a parent is involved in the abuse, confrontation at this point has no advantages and may have some disadvantages such as subsequent coercion placed on the child. The confrontation should be left to the **child abuse team** (involving trained police and social services) which will be activated. Where allegations have been made (for example against the father), the team will usually recommend he temporarily live elsewhere (e.g. with relatives) while investigations proceed. Most will comply.

- The child may need to be admitted to the paediatric ward (e.g. non-accidental injury suspected in casualty).

- Other agencies such as paediatricians, NSPCC or child mental health **risk assessment teams** may need to be involved. Investigations such as X-rays may be necessary.

- **Clear, contemporaneous documentation is important**.

- Social services will organise a **case conference**. The child's name may be placed on the **child**

abuse register. Careful assessment of risk is necessary and includes past history and the ability of the parent or parents to **accept responsibility** for their actions, **collusion** by the partner and so on. There may be a conclusion that the child is too much at risk to return home and the child will need to be taken into care, although efforts will be made to keep the child within the family when safe.

- There will be a need for discussions about the timing of any therapy. Initial therapeutic work may centre around **here and now** issues, for example **preparation for court**. Subsequent therapy should be tailored to the needs of the child.

- Individual or group therapy may be beneficial, and family therapy or parental counselling may be necessary. Minimise negative effects of abuse.

- Support the non-abusing carer.

Individual work

- Careful consideration of the sex of therapist.

- Allow ventilation of feelings and discussion of abuse. Acknowledge/validate their experiences.

- Clarify confusing issues and assess psychological disturbance.

- Teach self-protection. Inform/educate. Empower child.

- Address guilt/responsibility issues for being abused (e.g. enjoyment of some aspects of abuse, why they couldn't stop it, positive feelings towards abuser).

- Address fears (for example fear of homosexuality in male sexual abuse).

- Carer needs to be warned about possible negative behaviour during some stages of individual work.

Group therapy approaches

- Same gender groups are used. Offer a range of inputs including psychoeducational, cognitive, psychodynamic and supportive work.

- Some think it is best if there are male and female co-therapists.

- Keep carers informed. Carers' group may run simultaneously.

- Reduce isolation.

- Improve self-esteem.

- Educate.

- Severe acting out may hamper groups.

Parent training (secondary prevention)

- **Psychoeducational techniques** may be useful in training parents about safety, danger, hygiene, normal development and health. Unrealistic expectations may be challenged and appropriate responses (such as cognitive stimulation in infancy) may be encouraged.

- **Modelling approaches** have been used with community workers involved in guided parenting.

- **Cognitive behaviour therapy** may be useful, particularly with respect to self-control training in parents of young children. **Problem-solving skills** may allow parents to select alternative strategies to the previous abusive ones.

Other useful training techniques include:

- Anger control training.

- Stress management may be useful.

- Contingency management techniques (behaviour therapy).

Note. At least 50% of families where educational interventions have been attempted will go on abusing their children.[9]

Family therapy (see family therapy section of this chapter)

- Address secrecy/denial/disbelief.

- Assess functioning/support.

- Address siblings' needs/family response.

- Encourage support and openness.

- Encourage protection of members.

Other issues

- Consequences of legal system.
  - (i) the conflicts of therapy alongside evidence.
  - (ii) the effects of anxiety/stress, especially when there are court delays or cross-examination and the need for court preparation.
  - (iii) the consequences of the case not going to court/conviction not achieved/light sentence if convicted.

- Help for foster families.

- Treatment for abusers.

- Supervision for therapists.

Practical Treatments in Child Psychiatry

Child psychiatrists draw on a wide range of therapeutic interventions. These may be directed at the **child**, the **family**, the **parents** or the **child's environment** (through the education system or social services). Consultation and liaison with other disciplines is therefore an important part of work in child psychiatry. The following concentrates on interventions involving face to face contact.

Behaviour therapy

Great importance should be given to in-depth history taking at the planning stage, and **monitoring** of any response before, during and after treatment. The following strategies may be useful in a behavioural programme:

- **Positive reinforcement**: the desired behaviour is reinforced by praise or some other reward. This is a crucial part of all behaviour programmes in children. Subgroups of this (other than simple reward systems) include:

  (i)   **Shaping**: rewarding behaviours which increasingly **approximate** to the desired behaviour. Useful in children with learning disabilities.

  (ii) **DRO – Differential Reinforcement of Other behaviours**: reinforcing behaviours other than undesired ones. Used in hyperkinetic disorder, conduct disorder.

  (iii) **RIB – Reinforcing Incompatible Behaviour**: reinforcing behaviour which is incompatible with undesired behaviour. Useful in conduct disorder.

  (iv) **Differential reinforcement**: only reinforcing desired behaviour in the presence of particular (e.g. appropriate) circumstances/stimulus. Used in skills training.

- **Extinction**: withholding reward after inappropriate behaviour. For example by offering reduced attention after negative behaviour. (A sub-type of this is **time out from positive reinforcement**, where reinforcement is withdrawn for a particular length of time.)

- **Modelling**: the demonstration of behaviour by a trusted individual. This is useful for developing social skills, treating phobias, modelling positive behaviours (e.g. in conduct disorder) or to prevent fears developing (e.g. dentist).

- **Chaining** involves an adult allowing a child to successfully do part of an activity (e.g. doing up shirt buttons) and then initially helping them with the rest. The individual components of the behaviour are then added to a part at a time. May be used in social skills training and daily living skills training of children with learning difficulties.

- **Exposure, desensitisation and response prevention** techniques may be used to treat anxiety, obsessions, or phobias (see Chapter 5). **Flooding** and **implosion** (a variant of flooding involving imagination of severe anxiety-provoking situations) are rarely used with children.

- **Pad and bell** devices (several types available) are used in nocturnal enuresis where an alarm wakes the child early in the passing of urine. Understanding of the mechanism is not complete, but some involvement of classical and operant conditioning seems likely.

- **Antecedent modification** may be a helpful intervention if an antecedent is powerfully attached to a behaviour.

- **Contingency management** refers to a programme

which explores behaviour in some depth with **Antecedent, Behaviour and Consequence (ABC) diaries**. Many techniques such as **positive reinforcement** techniques may be used alongside techniques which aim to minimise behaviours.

- **Aversive techniques (punishments)** are punitive approaches **not much used** now in therapy but commonly found in families, including:

  (i) **Response costs** or fines for undesired behaviours.
  (ii) **Negative reinforcement**, which involves providing a mild aversive stimulus after negative behaviour and withholding it only when the desired behaviour is produced.
  (iii) **Covert sensitisation**, which uses imagined aversive stimuli, linked to unwanted behaviour.
  (iv) **Physical punishment**, which is commonly used in families but is thought to carry many risks. Apart from the risk of physical harm it can sometimes paradoxically offer attention from an adult which the child desires. It can therefore become a positive reinforcer to the negative behaviour which the adult set out to extinguish. It has a tendency to occur when the parent is angry or out of control and it may engender resentment in the child. If frequent, it teaches the child aggression as a central way of resolving conflicts.

Parent training

- This refers to psychoeducational approaches directed at improving the quality of parenting. Many authors have emphasised the point that parents do not have to be perfect, and that many different approaches may lead to successful child rearing (**good-enough** parenting).

- Parent training includes preparation such as Child Health courses in schools, and classes arranged through antenatal clinics. In America many community projects have targeted vulnerable sections of the community (for example single parents and low socio-economic groups) to improve parenting, with some success. Such courses may cover guidance in developmentally appropriate tasks and **behaviour management training**.

- **Other professionals** (e.g. midwives, health visitors, general practitioners, social workers and teachers) may all give advice at some time about the management of children.

- **Support groups** may target particular types of family such as single-parent families (e.g. "Gingerbread"), or specific conditions (e.g. hyperkinetic disorder). Other projects target parents who are under stress, providing emotional and practical support (e.g. "Homestart", "Newpin").

- There are many books on the subject that may be used as part of a self-help approach.

Family therapies

See later.

Group therapies

Many child mental health teams offer groups:

- **Psychoeducational**: social skills groups; survivor groups (e.g. disasters, bereavement, sexual abuse); physical illness groups (e.g. diabetes, asthma, cystic fibrosis).

- **Psychodynamic**: based on group processes and interpretations by the group therapist who observes pairing, scapegoating, fight/flight and dependence. Here and now. May be open or closed. Courses exist to give theoretical and practical training in this.

Other group therapies include:

- **Drama therapy**: simple drama therapy may involve using drama techniques to explore such things as boundaries and social skills; **psychodrama** involves acting out each individual's difficulties, using other members, and experimenting with roles and script changes. Interpretations and expression of feelings may be powerful, achieving insight and change.

Pharmacological treatments

- Medications such as minor tranquillisers or sedatives are little used by child psychiatrists. For example, sleep problems in toddlers are more likely to be treated by behaviour therapy, parental advice and support than drugs such as vallergan.

- There is little support for the use of anticonvulsants in behaviour-disordered children with non-specific EEG abnormalities in the absence of seizures.

Treatment of enuresis

- Behaviour therapy is largely preferred.

- Drugs are sometimes used as an adjunct but relapse is common after stopping.

- Tricyclics may be used in the short term (usually imipramine). The efficacy is not produced by the anticholinergic effects.

- Desmopressin (anti-diuretic hormone) may be given at bedtime.

Treatment of hyperkinetic disorder

- Methylphenidate, dexamphetamine (controlled drugs) and pemoline are all stimulants which have been shown to be useful in hyperkinetic disorder. They have definite short-term benefits.

- Methylphenidate reduces overactivity, improves concentration and reduces aggressive behaviour.

- There is less evidence about longer-term and educational effects and it is less useful in children with severe learning difficulties.

- 60–70% of children will respond; 25% not responding to one drug will respond to an alternative.

- Important to make clear that drug prescribing goes hand in hand with other interventions, particularly **educational interventions** and **behaviour therapy**.

- Euphoriant effects have not been reported below teenage years (no problems with abuse by child).

- The side-effect profile is large (mainly anorexia, sleep disturbance, reduced growth rate whilst on it, headaches, abdominal pains), therefore careful discussion with parents is required (informed consent). Drug holidays recommended to facilitate growth spurts.

Some other drugs have been suggested but not widely used:

- Imipramine, clonidine and less commonly haloperidol, chlorpromazine, moclobamide, fluoxetine and levodopa/carbidopa.

Treatment of depression in children

- Tricyclics are used in severe depression in children over 10–12. They appear less effective than in adults.

- Always given in conjunction with other interventions (e.g. psychotherapy).

- Tricyclics are not usually useful in school refusal.

Treatment of schizophrenia and manic-depressive psychosis

As for adult treatment.

Treatment of autism and related disorders

- Short course of treatment is sometimes helpful as an adjunct, e.g. haloperidol for aggression.

- Many other drugs have been suggested but not widely used (e.g. stimulants, beta-blockers, vitamin B6 and magnesium). No good studies have shown any dramatic benefits with drugs.

Treatment of complex or severe tics and Gilles de la Tourette syndrome

- Haloperidol (or pimozide) can reduce tic activity in small doses. It is not curative and there may be a rebound of symptoms when stopped.

Individual psychotherapy

- Child psychotherapy usually refers to **psycho-dynamic psychotherapy**. Containment, understanding the child through the relationship, interpretations and transference all play a part in treating emotional disorders. Many clinicians would like to see more studies showing effectiveness.

- **Play therapy** uses play as a medium, and art therapists may use a variety of ways of allowing the child to express themselves in the context of the psychotherapeutic relationship. Interpretations and clarifications are made which are used in the therapy.

- Increasingly, **cognitive behavioural** approaches are also being used. This is useful for anxiety, depression, anger and aggression.

- Supportive and bereavement counselling may also be offered at an individual level.

- Individual therapy is less useful in children who have severe learning difficulties or problems with symbolic thought.

- Ensure that teachers and parents acknowledge and support changes to maintain any positive gains made.

Dyad work and marital therapy

Any dyad within the family can be seen together. This may have benefits for child and family, but will not be covered here.

The role of diet

- Exclusion diets are still sometimes used, but not commonly by child mental health workers.

- Tartrazine and salicylates have **not** been shown to be significant causes of problem behaviour by controlled trials, although they may be relevant in a minority of cases.

- Some clinicians report benefit from exclusion diets which re-introduce and therefore identify particular foodstuffs (e.g. wheatflour, caffeine).

Day patient units

Useful for assessment and close monitoring (e.g. autism spectrum disorders), and when more intensive treatment is necessary (e.g. school refusal, severe soiling).

In-patient units

- Used for assessment and treatment.

- Important to continue working with the rest of the family during the admission.

Note. Children's Units and Adolescent Units are not available in all districts. Admission is avoided if possible, especially with children. They are used when out-patient therapy fails or the clinical presentation is severe (e.g. in psychosis, eating disorders or school refusal).

Family Therapy

Family therapy seeks to identify dysfunctional processes within a family system and generate healthy change. Most models and therapeutic approaches draw upon **systems theory**[10] which highlights the fact that each family is a system with sub-systems within it (e.g. parents, children). Identifiable patterns of communication are observable. It recognises the key notion of circular, not just linear, causality within systems (e.g. positive feedback, negative feedback, and interactional effects within relationships). Many clinicians do family work without calling it family therapy, and for this reason some authors draw a distinction between this (**informal family therapy**) and **formal family therapy**, described below.

Formal family therapy[11]

- A team approach is used which consists of a variety of professionals from different disciplines (e.g. psychiatrists, psychologists, social workers, community psychiatric nurses, occupational therapists, child psychotherapists, etc.).

- The team operates behind a one-way mirror (or video link) with one or two therapists in front with the family.

- Five parts to organisation of therapy were first described by the Milan School (see later), but are now very widely used:
  (i)   Pre-session hypothesising.
  (ii) Session with family.
  (iii) Team break and discussion of family and session.
  (iv) Feedback to family.
  (v)   Post-session discussion about family responses.

- Various methods are used for the team to communicate observations and ideas to the therapist/s during the session. These include phoning through, knocking on the door, an electronic earpiece, and taking a break.

Uses of family therapy

- Widely used in child mental health teams throughout the United Kingdom, and beyond.

- Useful where family dysfunction is identified and appears amenable to treatment.

- Where family (or members of it) act as maintaining factor(s) for the problem or symptom of the child, or where the symptom in the child is an **expression of family dysfunction**.

- Various "schools" of family therapy use different ways of achieving change.

Schools of Family Therapy

- Most therapists use techniques derived from different schools.

- All accept the need to engage family.

- Most acknowledge some transgenerational factors.

- All accept different cultural influences on family life.

Structural family therapy (Minuchin)[12]

Salvador Minuchin is an Argentinian-born psychoanalyst working in the United States. He popularised the use of a one-way screen and observing the therapist.

Structure of the family is defined by:

- Role of each member/interplay of roles.

- Hierarchies in the family.

- Coalitions/alliances (**alignments**).

- Family "rules" and "games".

- Boundaries.

- Stability (**coherence**).

- Flexibility.

- Therapist **accommodating** to **join with** (be accepted by) the family.

- Assessment of structure and sub-systems.

- Identification of dysfunction.

The therapist is particularly looking for:

- Overinvolvement (**enmeshment**).

- Underinvolvement (**detachment**).

- Negative feelings from one relationship projected or expressed onto third party within family (**triangulation, detouring**)

Tasks are set, and techniques employed, to address the family dysfunction:

- **Unbalance** (by taking sides).

- Disturb alliances and coalitions.

- Alter structure, for example by:
  - (i) Returning power and responsibility to parents.
  - (ii) Establishing clear generational hierarchies.
  - (iii) Establishing honest, open communication.
  - (iv) Reducing scapegoating.
  - (v) Disrupting dysfunctional interactions (suggesting alternatives, etc.).

Strategic family therapy (Madanes[13] and others, e.g. Jay Haley)

- Essentially a non-critical approach.

- Symptom or goal is made the target. Desired outcome agreed with the family.

- Less attention to underlying dysfunction.

- Directive approach geared to empower family or members of it.

- Emphasis on the **meaning** of the symptom within the family.

Broad-minded strategies or techniques employed:

- Interpreting.

- Task setting.

- Relabelling/**positively reframing** (e.g. **positively connoting content** or **context** of behaviour).

- Behaviour therapy techniques.

- Confrontation.

- Externalising problems (e.g. *"the sneaky pooh"* of encopresis).

- **Paradoxical interventions** may increase the resolve of the family (e.g. prescribing the symptom, predicting failure or relapse).

Milan School (Selvini Palazzoli[14] and others)

- Not as directive. Has a psychoanalytic background.

- Less emphasis on restructuring by strategies.

- More emphasis on family achieving **insight** by exploring each others positions and exposing dysfunctional family patterns.

- Insight produces desire to change.

Use of techniques during therapy:

- Neutrality of the therapist.

- Recognition of **circularity** in systems (e.g. positive and negative feedback to behaviour and interactions).

- **Triangular questioning**, e.g. using a third person to discuss interactions of other two. This acts as a powerful feedback for use in sessions.

- Paradox (see above).

- Positive reframing/connotation (see above).

Other approaches

Various other schools have developed from existing schools:

- **Brief solution focused family therapy**[15] involves concentrating on the problem presented by the family, and being specific about the goal and target of therapy. Strategies and tasks are designed which aim to achieve the goals efficiently, without necessarily seeking family insight into problems.

- **Family tree construction**, to elicit important information about family relationships and transgenerational issues.

- Allowing the family to **watch the team deliberations** about the family. This can give the family clearer insight into how they are perceived. Careful attention must be paid by the team to how observations and thoughts are expressed, to achieve benefit for the family.

- Having family members behind the screen directing the therapists in what questions are asked. This is useful where secrets paralyse the family.

Effectiveness of family therapy

Studies show usefulness in:

- Conduct-disordered children.

- Eating disorders.

- Amelioration of family distress.

- Improving family functioning in chronic physical illness.

More methodologically sound studies are needed. Overall, family therapy is useful and worthwhile,[16] although the specific mechanisms of success are not clear from the research available.

Key points

- 0.4% of children under 18 are on a child protection register.

- Child abuse has important short- and long-term effects on a child's development.

- Assessment and treatment should be sensitively handled, holistic and tailored to the particular situation.

- Treatments in child mental care are wide ranging and multidisciplinary in style.

- Family therapy draws heavily upon systems theory, and various approaches are used to seek change within the family.

- Family therapy has been shown to be effective, although more research is needed.

References

[1] Finkelhor D, Korbin J (1988). Child abuse as an international issue. *Child Abuse and Neglect*, **12**, 2–24.

[2] Thompson A E, Kaplan C A (1996). Childhood emotional abuse. *British Journal of Psychiatry*, **168**, 143–148.

[3] Kempe C H, Silverman F M, Steele B F, Droegmueller W, Silver H K (1962). The battered child syndrome. *Journal of the American Medical Association*, **181**, 4–11.

[4] Baker A W, Duncan S P (1985) Child sexual abuse: a study of prevalence in Great Britain. *Child Abuse and Neglect*, **9,** 457–467.

[5] Meadow R (1977). Munchausen syndrome by proxy. The hinterland of child abuse. *Lancet*, **ii**, 343–345.

[6] Finkelhor D (1988). The trauma of child sexual abuse: two models. In *Lasting Effects of Child Sexual Abuse*, (eds) Wyatt G E, Powell G J. London: Sage, pp. 61–82.

[7] Summitt R C (1983). The child sexual abuse accommodation syndrome. *Child Abuse and Neglect*, **7**, 177–193.

[8] Department of Health (1988). *Working Together: A Guide to the Arrangements for Interagency Co-operation for the Protection of Children from Abuse*. London: HMSO.

[9] Cohn A H, Daro D (1987). Is treatment too late? What ten years of evaluative research tells us. *Child Abuse and Neglect*, **11**, 433–442.

[10] Von Bertalanffy L (1968). *General Systems Theory: Foundations, Development, Application*. New York: Braziller.

[11] Barker P (1992). *Basic Family Therapy*. London: Blackwell Scientific Publications.

[12] Minuchin S (1974). *Families and Family Therapy*. Massachusetts: Harvard University Press.

[13] Madanes C (1981). *Strategic Family Therapy*. San Francisco: Jossey Bass.

[14] Selvini Palazzoli M, Boscolo L, Cecchin G, Prata G (1980). Hypothesising-circularity-neutrality: three guidelines for the conductor of the session. *Family Process*, **19**, 3–12.

[15] De Shazer S, Berg I K, Lipchik E, Nunnally E, Molnar A, Gingerich Weiner-Davis M (1986). Brief therapy: focused solution development. *Family Process*, **25**, 207–222.

[16] Markus E, Lange A, Pettigrew T (1990). Effectiveness of family therapy: a meta-analysis. *Journal of Family Therapy*, **12**, 205–221.

Chapter 8

Molecular genetics in psychiatry

Nick Brindle

Psychiatric disorders have neither a purely genetic nor environmental aetiology, but are a result of complex interactions between these factors. Disentangling the relative contributions of these components relies, to some extent, on quantitative genetic analyses such as family, twin and adoption studies. For example, it is known that schizophrenia may cluster in families, but it is only through the combination of family, twin and adoption studies that a genetic vulnerability can be ascertained.

The purpose of this chapter is to highlight important aspects of molecular genetics. You will need to supplement this by reading other accounts of molecular genetic research including revising the terminology used, and especially the research involving twin and family studies.

Having established a genetic contribution for a given disorder it is now possible, using the rapidly developing technology of molecular genetics, to locate and identify disease-causing genes and to gain some understanding of the underlying pathological mechanisms. The route from genotype to identifying, cloning and characterising a disease gene requires a number of complex steps. First, the generation of genetic markers, then performance of linkage analysis and finally positional cloning in order to identify the site of the disease-causing gene.

Molecular Genetic Techniques Used in the Isolation of Mutated Genes

Restriction Fragment Length Polymorphisms (RFLPs)

- **Polymorphisms** (different forms of the same allele) in the human genome may be due to **natural variation** in the population or result from either an inherited or somatic **mutation**.

- **Restriction enzymes** are nucleases that have the ability to cleave deoxyribonucleic acid (DNA). There are over a hundred of such enzymes known, and each one recognises a specific sequence of DNA – commonly four to eight base pairs in length. For example, the restriction enzyme Not1 has an eight base pair recognition motif, GCGGC-CGC, and will sever DNA wherever this sequence is found. Restriction enzymes are used widely in molecular cloning and simplify the analysis of DNA. Any change to a nucleotide sequence can destroy or create an enzyme recognition site. This will be shown by a different pattern of restriction fragments on gel electrophoresis. These are called **Restriction Fragment Length Polymorphisms (RFLPs)**.

- RFLPs are detected by digestion of DNA by one or more restriction enzymes, to produce fragments of different lengths. These are separated by **agarose gel electrophoresis**. DNA migrates through the gel at a rate inversely proportional to its molecular size. It can then be visualised and photographed by staining with ethidium bromide, a dye that intercalates into the double stranded DNA and fluoresces under ultraviolet light.

Southern blotting

The technique of Southern blotting is used to compare the gene structure of different individuals. It may be used to identify single nucleotide base pair alterations, as well as being able to detect more gross abnormalities such as gene deletions. An easily identified **probe** (e.g. one that is radioactive) is used to bind to its **complementary DNA sequence**.

- The DNA is digested with a series of **restriction enzymes**. Fragments are separated by size using agarose gel electrophoresis and then transferred to a membrane that binds nucleic acids. The hydrogen bonds between the two complementary DNA strands are then broken to produce single strands by treatment with sodium hydroxide. Labelled DNA complementary to the region of interest will bind to this sequence on the Southern blot and can be subsequently visualised.

- **Methods of labelling DNA** include the use of radioactivity, biotin, enymes and fluorescent markers.

Northern blotting

Ribonucleic acid (RNA) transcripts, such as messenger RNA (mRNA), can be characterised using the technique of Northern blotting. The principles of RNA separation, transfer, probe hybridisation and detection are similar to Southern blotting for DNA.

DNA cloning

This is a process of generating **multiple identical copies of a DNA sequence** of interest for labelling, sequencing, mutation and expression studies. Fragments of DNA can be cloned using a variety of vector/host systems. The choice will depend on a number of different factors such as the size of DNA to be cloned, the requirement for cloning, efficiency of the cloning procedure, generation of single stranded DNA for sequencing and DNA mutation, need for expression of protein, etc.

- The first stage in molecular cloning involves the construction of **DNA libraries** from genomic DNA or cDNA (complementary DNA) which is manufactured enzymically from mRNA. Genomic libraries representing the entire genome are prepared by digesting DNA with a restriction enzyme to generate large DNA fragments. These fragments are cloned or ligated into vector DNA.

- There are **four major types of vector: plasmid, bacteriophage, cosmid and yeast artificial chromosomes** (**YACs**), each with different properties. Generally plasmid and bacteriophage vectors are used for cloning relatively smaller fragments of DNA such as cDNA, whereas cosmids and YACs are used for cloning much larger genomic fragments of DNA. A map of the human genome has been constructed using YACs.

After constructing a library, the recombinant clone of interest must be identified and purified. For libraries contained in bacteria, the library is plated out and hybridised to a radiolabelled probe, complementary to the sequence of interest. Colonies that demonstrate a positive signal are picked and regrown. By repeating the plating, probing and picking procedure, clones can be isolated that contain at least part of the gene of interest.

Fluorescent *In-Situ* Hybridisation (FISH)

- FISH combines the specificity of molecular genetics with traditional cytogenetics. It is a technique whereby a biotin or digoxigenin labelled nucleic acid probe is hybridised to either metaphase chromosomes or to cells. The probes used are generally DNA such as labelled yeast artificial chromosomes **(YACs)**.

- Visualisation of hybridised probes is by fluorescence microscopy. Applications of FISH include identification of marker chromosomes, translocation breakpoints and characterisation of chromosomal rearrangements.

Polymerase Chain Reaction (PCR)

- PCR is an extraordinarily powerful technique and has a great many applications in both research and in the routine diagnostic laboratory. It is sensitive, potentially capable of amplifying DNA or RNA from a single cell. It is a highly specific test, technically very simple to perform and can be used to amplify DNA from many samples, simultaneously.

- The specificity of the PCR is determined by the sequence of the oligonucleotide primers that are complementary to each end of the sequence to be amplified. To amplify RNA transcripts, a preliminary step occurs in which RNA is converted to single stranded DNA using a **reverse transcriptase** (RNA dependent DNA polymerase). This procedure is known as **RT-PCR**.

- With each cycle of the procedure, two new strands of DNA are generated from the one originally present.

- The cycle is repeated, with the **amount of DNA doubling each time**. Normally 20–40 cycles are performed in automated thermocycling devices producing a 10^5–10^6 **amplification of target DNA**

within a few hours. Amplified products are then analysed by agarose or acrylamide gel electrophoresis and subsequent staining with ethidium bromide.

- **DNA generated by PCR** can also be used for DNA sequence analysis, characterising mutations, genomic mapping and in creating site directed mutations that can be **used to investigate gene structure and function**. PCR is often used to identify a specific mutation or polymorphism in a gene that causes an inherited disease, or for analysis of genes in which mutations are suspected but the precise location of the mutation is not known.

Linkage analysis

- Linkage analysis is generally the first step on the road to positional cloning of a disease gene. **The procedure is based upon the identification of disease genes by way of their proximity to genetic marker loci**.

- Linkage analysis can be used for **single gene defects** where a clearly defined pattern of inheritance is apparent. It is most useful in analysing genetic diseases transmitted in a simple Mendelian fashion, i.e. autosomal dominant/recessive or sex linked. It requires definition of certain genetic parameters, such as the mode of transmission.

- When analysing complex multifactorial genetic traits displaying non-Mendelian patterns of inheritance the **sib pair analysis** form of linkage analysis can be used. This relies on determining shared alleles between pairs of affected siblings. Linkage to a disease susceptibility locus is demonstrated in a particular region of a chromosome if siblings share certain alleles more than is expected by chance.

- The **recombination fraction (θ)** is a measure of the likelihood that a crossover will occur between two loci during meiosis, and therefore **a measure of the genetic distance between loci**. A θ value of 0.5 indicates that two loci are not linked. When assessing for linkage a series of likelihood ratios are calculated for different values of θ (from 0 to 0.5) and expressed as the **logarithm of the odds (lod score or Z)**. Significant linkage is considered when the **lod score is greater than three**. A score of −2 discounts linkage. Multipoint analysis is a more sophisticated technique that enables greater precision by examining segregation of alleles at a number of closely adjacent loci.

- In order to calculate lod scores, various genetic parameters must be specified. Often these parameters cannot be stated with certainty and an incorrect specification may act to reduce the lod score. In contrast, multiple test effects arising from analysis of a range of genetic models can artificially inflate the lod score. Fortunately, modern computer software can correct for some of these errors. This is highly relevant to psychiatry where disease definition may be a major problem.

- **Microsatellite DNA** consists of repeats (typically 15–30 repeats) of small segments of DNA, two, three or four base pairs in size that appear to be evenly distributed throughout the genome. It has been estimated that there are between 50 000 and 100 000 of these microsatellite repeats distributed throughout the human genome occurring on average once in every 100 000 base pairs. **Construction of a high resolution physical map of the human genome has only been possible since the advent of microsatellite markers**. They provide a means of indirectly tracking genes necessary for linkage analysis.

Genetic markers used in linkage analysis

- Variable number of tandem repeats (VNTRs).

- Microsatellite repeat sequences, e.g. (CA)n repeats.

- Restriction fragment length polymorphisms (RFLPs).

Strategies to help in pin-pointing likely positions of disease-causing genes

- Screening individuals for **cytogenetic abnormalities** such as insertions, deletions or translocations that co-segregate with a mental disorder may indicate a region of interest.

- The objective of the **candidate gene approach** is to identify polymorphisms in genes that have been implicated in the pathogenesis of a disorder, e.g. the dopamine receptor genes in schizophrenia.

- If there are no cytogenetic abnormalities or suitable candidate genes, a whole genome search attempting to link disease locus to markers of known chromosomal localisation is necessary.

Positional cloning

Once linkage has been established to a particular region of a chromosome using linkage analysis techniques, the next stage in positional cloning requires the construction of **a high resolution physical map of the region** followed by identification of candidate genes. An overlapping YAC set of DNA clones of the disease gene locus is then constructed. Genes can be isolated from individual YACs and analysed for mutations in affected families.

Stages in positional cloning

- Accurately define phenotype.

- Perform linkage analysis.

- Search for more tightly linked markers.

- Construct high resolution physical map of region.

- Search for expressed genes in the region.

- Look for mutations in candidate genes.

- Confirm relationship between mutation and disease.

Inherited Psychiatric Disease

There are a number of problems when applying the procedures described above to clinical psychiatry. Linkage analysis is extremely useful in detecting **single** gene disorders, but many psychiatric disorders such as schizophrenia and the affective disorders are **multifactorial**. Different variants may be characterised by different genotypes, and different environmental interactions. In the case of later onset conditions, such as Alzheimer's disease, there may not be many affected relatives surviving – especially affected parents.

- There has been substantial progress in improving the reliability and consensus of psychiatric diagnoses. However, limitations of diagnostic validity remain because of the absence of ratifying criteria. This may limit the power of genetic techniques.

- **Inaccuracies in the definition of the phenotype** (equivalent here to the psychiatric diagnosis) arise from several sources. Errors may be introduced by conditions that overlap diagnostic categories such as the schizoaffective states. Furthermore, it is also unclear exactly which conditions should be included in the definition of spectrum disorders. Spectrum disorders arise from variation in the phenotypic expression of a gene (expressivity). Examples include schizotypy which is considered to represent a variation in the expressivity of the schizophrenic genotype.

- Improvements need to be made in the collection and categorisation of patient information, to increase the possibility of detecting linkage in multifactorial psychiatric conditions. Use of sib pair analysis, improvement in the clinical characterisation, statistical analysis and greater consideration of the gene and environment interaction should improve the prospects of success.

- Analysis of larger sample sizes, which is certainly possible with the current trend toward collaborative studies, is a major step forward.

Schizophrenia

There are strong indications for a genetic predisposition to schizophrenia despite mounting evidence for a neurodevelopmental aetiology to the disorder. Perinatal insults may interact with a genetic susceptibility to influence the development of the disorder. Studies have not defined a mode of inheritance, though a variety of models have been proposed, e.g. an **oligogenetic** (several genes contribute) **model with environmental effects**.

Through identifying cytogenetic abnormalities, a segmental duplication of a region of **chromosome 5q** has been noted to co-segregate with schizophrenia in some families.[1] (In cytogenetic terminology, chromosomes are denoted into **short arm (p) and**

long arm (q) joined at the centromere. The arms are subdived into regions, bands and sub-bands from the **centromere** to the **telomere**, or end of the chromosome. **Therefore 14q24.3 denotes the long arm of chromosome 14, region 2, band 4, sub-band 3**.)

- A further study showed linkage between schizophrenia and an RFLP in the **5q region**,[2] though this has not subsequently been replicated.

- Attention has also been directed to a region of **chromosome 11q** because several genes which have been implicated in the aetiology of schizophrenia map to this region. These include the dopamine D2 receptor gene, porphobilinogen deaminase gene and the tyrosinase gene. In addition several families have been reported in which a translocation and a psychotic illness co-segregate. However, comprehensive screens of this region have failed to demonstrate linkage.[3]

- The dopamine hypothesis would tend to suggest that at least indirectly a functional abnormality in one of the cerebral dopaminergic systems con-tributes to the symptoms of schizophrenia. The dopamine receptor genes are therefore potential **candidate genes** for investigation. There are now five different dopamine receptors identified (D1–D5). With the exception of an association between schizophrenia and homozygosity at a D3 receptor locus, linkage appears to have been excluded in the remaining receptor genes.[4, 5]

- The velocardiofacial syndrome is a chromosomal disorder caused by microdeletions in the region of **chromosome 22q11**. Individuals present with cleft palate, facial defects and cardiac malformations. It is also associated with psychiatric disorders in approximately 10% of patients, most commonly a chronic paranoid schizophrenic illness. This would suggest that a locus in the region may be involved in the aetiology of schizophrenia in at least some cases.

- **A pseudoautosomal region** of the sex chromosomes has been suggested as being linked.[6] Again these findings are yet to be successfully replicated.

- Candidate domains identified by genome wide searches have included regions **on chromosomes 4, 14, 15 and 22**.[7] More recently workers have reported a lod score of three for linkage to a **chromosome 6** marker close to the SCA1 locus, though further corroboration has not been forthcoming.[8]

- Alterations in other neurotransmitter systems have been implicated in the pathogenesis of schizophrenia. One group has identified a γ amino butyric acid (GABA) receptor gene variant transmitted from an unaffected father to two affected siblings.[9] The pathological significance of this is unclear.

The available evidence and the inconsistencies of the linkage analysis approach **suggests a non-Mendelian pattern of inheritance in schizophrenia**. However, improvements in the design of linkage studies in the future may facilitate progress and identify genes of importance in this condition.

Affective disorders

- The aetiological complexity of affective disorders make these difficult conditions to investigate using linkage analysis. There appears to be an important genetic contribution though, as in the case of schizophrenia, it is yet to be clearly defined.

- Early linkage studies concentrated on **chromosome 11p**.[10] They described close linkage of DNA markers to a locus conferring predisposition to manic depressive illness in the Old-order Amish in Pennsylvania.

- Other studies including those in Iceland, the United States and Great Britain failed to confirm this result.[11] The enzyme tyrosine hydroxylase, which catalyses the rate limiting step in the synthesis of catecholamines, maps to **chromosome 11p** and was proposed as a possible candidate gene with regard to the affective psychoses. Although associations of polymorphisms in this gene in affective psychosis had been reported, these findings were not confirmed when the study was subsequently repeated on other pedigrees. (Examination of other candidate genes such as those for the dopamine D2 and D3 receptors and scrutiny of classical markers such as the HLA system have not revealed any linkage.)

- Other studies have been focused on the **X chromosome** because of the supposed excess of female sufferers of these conditions. For example, a linkage between colour blindness and bipolar affective disorder, and linkage between a potential locus and the **factor IX gene in the Xq27 region** have been suggested.[12]

- Associations between markers in the monoamine oxidase A gene and bipolar affective disorder have been noted but not verified.

Alzheimer's disease

- The main neuropathological features of Alzheimer's disease are **extracellular amyloid plaques** and **intracellular neurofibrillary tangles**.

- The major component of amyloid plaques is an insoluble protein fragment called **amyloid β protein (Aβ)**.

- Aβ arises from proteolytic processing of a larger protein, the **amyloid precursor protein (APP)**.

- **Processing of APP can occur by two pathways**. The first is catalysed by a putative α secretase and results in a product that does not contain all the AβP sequence and does not precipitate to form amyloid. The second pathway, via an endosomal/lysosomal pathway, results in the production of Aβ and subsequent amyloid deposition.

- The **amyloid cascade hypothesis** supports the view that the deposition of AβP is the causative agent of Alzheimer's disease, and that the other pathological features and dementia follow as a result of its precipitation.[13]

- The function of APP is not yet known, though a number of potential roles have been ascribed to this protein. It may be a cell surface receptor, or have a role in neuronal repair mechanisms.

- Neurofibrillary tangles consist of dense unbranched filaments called **paired helical filaments (PHF)**. The major protein of PHFs is the microtubule-associated τ (tau) **protein**. τ protein becomes abnormally phosphorylated in Alzheimer's disease and aggregates to form PHFs.[14]

- There is little evidence that τ alone is sufficient to cause Alzheimer's disease, though an **interaction between τ and AβP may play a role in plaque and tangle formation.**[15]

Familial Alzheimer's disease

Alzheimer's disease is known to cluster in families. There is **a threefold increase in incidence in first degree relatives of affected individuals**. Familial Alzheimer's disease is now well recognised, and over 100 families have been reported in which the disease shows an **autosomal dominant** pattern of inheritance. There are four known chromosomal loci linked to familial Alzheimer's disease in different pedigrees: **chromosomes 21q21, 19q13.2, 14q24 and 1q31–34** (familial Alzheimer's disease 1–4, respectively).

- **Mutations in the APP gene** are found at the familial Alzheimer's disease 1 locus on **chromosome 21q21**.[16] Such mutations are rare and responsible for only a small proportion of cases of presenile dementia.

- No mutations have been reported in "sporadic" cases of Alzheimer's disease. (The mutations may alter the capability of the APP to be metabolised by the "correct" pathway, and so direct degradation via the amyloidogenic route.)

- The almost universal incidence of Alzheimer's disease type pathology in **Down's syndrome sufferers**[17] surviving past the age of 30 may reflect a dosage effect of the APP gene caused by the trisomy 21, although other genes may be involved.

- **Apolipoprotein E** is thought to be involved in many processes in the central nervous system such as protein processing. There are three alleles, E2, E3 and E4 of the apolipoprotein E (apo E) gene at the familial Alzheimer's disease 2 locus on chromosome 19q13.[18] The E4 allele is associated with an increased relative risk of late onset Alzheimer's disease, and inheritance of two apo E4 alleles can decrease the mean age of onset by 15 years.

- Approximately 75% of families segregating Alzheimer's disease demonstrate linkage to the familial Alzheimer's disease 3 locus found at chromosome 14q24. A number of mutations in a gene (**presenilin 1 or PS-1**) from this region have been noted to be consistently mutated in **chromosome-14**-linked affected family members.[19] These mutations result in amino acid changes in the protein and have not been observed in unaffected family members. (PS-1 is thought to be an integral membrane protein.)

- A gene closely resembling the PS-1 gene was cloned at the familial Alzheimer's disease 4 locus on chromosome 1. This gene, **PS-2**, is mutated in affected members of the Volga German Alzheimer's disease pedigrees and in some other kindreds.[20]

- **There have been dramatic advances in the field of Alzheimer's disease genetics**. Now the presenilin genes have been identified, further work is necessary to investigate the proteins that they encode and their role in the pathogenesis of familial Alzheimer's disease. Though the sporadic form of the disease is likely to be aetiologically more heterogeneous, such impetus may add to the understanding of this devastating and prevalent disease.

Trinucleotide repeat diseases

Several inherited neurological diseases are now known to be associated with expansion of "unstable trinucleotide repeats". These repeats demonstrate the phenomenon of **anticipation**; that is, they increase in size over successive generations associated with worsening of the disease phenotype. **There are several disorders of this type**:

- **Fragile X** syndrome (the most common of these disorders; repeat sequence is CGG).
- **FRAXE** mental retardation.
- **Huntington's** disease.
- Spinocerebellar ataxia type 1 (SCA 1).
- X-linked spinal and bulbar muscular atrophy.
- Myotonic dystrophy.

Fragile X:

- The Fragile X syndrome (FRAX-A) is a common cause **of moderate to severe mental retardtion**, second in prevalence to Down's syndrome. The pattern of inheritance is unusual in that it can be transmitted by unaffected males (normal transmitting males) and carrier females may be mildly affected. The **Fragile X site is a non-staining band on the X chromosome which becomes evident when lymphocytes are grown in certain media**.

- There is an expanded CGG repeat in the first exon of the FMR-1 gene at the Fragile X site[21] in affected patients. There may be over 200 copies of this repeat sequence in sufferers compared with 6–54 in unaffected individuals.

- A PCR-based assay is now available to detect the mutations in the Fragile X syndrome (see above), though how the phenotype is produced because of this mutation is not yet known.

Huntington's disease (HD):

- Huntington's disease is an **autosomal dominant disorder with virtually 100% penetrance**. It is characterised by **chorea** and **dementia**, and is associated with a number of psychiatric manifestations – including paranoid psychosis.

- The mutation causing HD is a trinucleotide expansion in a gene called IT 15 on **chromosome 4q16.3**.[22] Unaffected individuals possess 11–34 copies of the CAG repeat sequence, whereas sufferers may possess 37–121 copies.

- The normal product of IT 15 is not known, but it may be a **regulatory protein**. Normal cellular function may be perturbed in HD, leading to neurodegeneration in a cell specific manner.

There remains a great deal to elucidate about the trinucleotide repeat diseases, not least the normal functioning of each of the disease genes, the mechanism of action of these mutations, and how they act in a cell specific manner. Such dynamic mutations may have a fundamental role in human genetics. A better understanding may lead to rational interventions to overcome the dysfunction.

Mental retardation

- Mental retardation is aetiologially heterogeneous, with a diversity of genetic and environmental factors playing a part.

- **Mild mental retardation** has traditionally been thought of as a **sub-cultural handicap** representing the lower end of the population distribution for IQ scores, dependent on an interplay between polygenic inheritance and social/educational disadvantage. Also, individuals without any definable cause of mental retardation are generally the more mildly affected. There has unfortunately been remarkably little interest in the genetics of this group, though there appears to be familial clustering and a high concordance in monozygotic twins.

- A broad division places mild mental retardation in the IQ score range of 50–70 and severe mental retardation in the 0–50 range.

- **Severe mental retardation** is considered to be pathological due to **specific disease processes**, such as:

  (i)   Genetic disorders.
  (ii) Congenital malformations.
  (iii) Perinatal injury.
  (iv) Infections.
  (v)   Inherited biochemical defects.

There is some evidence to support the distinction of mild and severe retardation on this basis, though the discrimination is to some extent **arbitrary** with a degree of overlap. One study found chromosomal abnormalities in 19% of mildly mentally retarded individuals.[23]

There are a large number of **single gene disorders** contributing to the severe end of the spectrum. Molecular genetics has been instrumental in mapping the chromosomal locations of the disease-causing genes, and in identifying pathological mutations (see Tables 8.1(a)–(d)).

It is worthwhile considering how the **advent of molecular genetics has contributed to the understanding and diagnosis of mental retardation** by mapping, cloning and basic molecular biological techniques. For instance, it has long been known that phenylketonuria (PKU) is due to deficiency of phenylalanine hydroxylase enzyme. As a result of the application of molecular genetic techniques, it is now appreciated that the gene is located on chromosome 12q24.1, and that 60 different mutations occurring in this enzyme, as well as mutations in dihydropterine reductase, may cause varying severity of the PKU phenotype.

Table 8.1(a) Chromosomal abnormalities

Chromosomal disorder	Chromosomal abnormality
Autosomal chromosomes	
Cri du chat	Partial deletion 5
Down's syndrome	Trisomy 21
Edward's syndrome	Trisomy 18
Patau's syndrome	Trisomy 13
Sex chromosomes	
Turner's syndrome	45 XO
Klinefelter's syndrome	47 XXY
XYY	XXY

Table 8.1(b) Examples of **autosomal recessive conditions** causing mental retardation

Disorder	Chromosomal location
Ataxia telengiectasia (Louis–Bar syndrome)	11q 22–q23
Hypertelorism (Grieg's syndrome)	—
Laurence Moon Biedl	—
Virchow–Seckel dwarf	—

Table 8.1(c) Examples of **autosomal dominant disorders** causing mental retardation

Disorder	Chromosomal location
Tuberose sclerosis	Type 1 9q33–q34
Acrocephalo-syndactyly (Apert's syndrome)	—
Mandibulo-facial dysostosis	5q31.3–q33.3

Table 8.1(d) Examples of **inborn errors of metabolism** causing mental retardation

Disorder	Mode of inheritance
Protein metabolism	
Hartnup disease	Autosomal recessive
Histidinaemia	—
Homocystinuria	—
Maple syrup disease	—
Phenylketonuria	—

continued . . .

Table 8.1(d) Examples of **inborn errors of metabolism** causing mental retardation (continued)

Lipid metabolism
Gaucher's disease	Autosomal recessive
Niemann Pick's disease	—
Tay–Sach's disease	—

Carbohyrate metabolism
Galactosaemia	Autosomal recessive

Connective tissue
Hurler's syndrome	Autosomal recessive
Hunter's syndrome	X-linked

Other X-linked disorders
Nephrogenic diabetes insipidus
Occulocerebral degeneration (Norrie's syndrome)
Lowe's syndrome

Suggested Further Reading

Brock D H J (1993). *Molecular Genetics for the Clinician*. Cambridge: Cambridge University Press.

Drugs and Therapeutics Bulletin (1996). A glossary of molecular genetics. *Drugs and Therapeutics Bulletin*, **34** (2), 15–16.

McGuffin P *et al*. (1994). *Seminars in Psychiatric Genetics*. London: The Royal College of Psychiatrists.

Thapar A, Gottesman I, Owen M *et al*. (1994). The genetics of mental retardation. *British Journal of Psychiatry*, **164**, 747–758.

References

[1] McGillivray B C, Bassett A S *et al*. (1990). Familial 5q11.2-q13.3 segmental duplication cosegregating with multiple anomalies including schizophrenia. *American Journal of Medical Genetics*, **35**, 10–13.

[2] Sherrington R, Brynjolfsson J, Petursson H *et al*. (1988). Localisation of a susceptibility locus for schizophrenia on chromosome 5. *Nature*, **336**, 164–167.

[3] Gill M, McGuffin P, Parfitt E *et al*. (1993). A linkage study of schizophrenia with DNA markers from the long arm of chromosome 11. *Psychological Medicine*, **23**, 27–44.

[4] Coon H, Byerley W, Holik J *et al*. (1993). Linkage analysis of schizophrenia with five dopamine receptor genes in nine pedigrees. *American Journal of Human Genetics*, **52**, 327–334.

[5] Crocq, M A, Byerley W, Hoik J *et al.* (1992). Association between schizophrenia and homozygosity at the Dopamine D3 receptor gene. *American Journal of Human Genetics*, **52**, 327–334.

[6] Collinge J, DeLisi L E, Boccio A *et al.* (1991). Evidence for a pseudo-autosomal locus for schizophrenia using the method of affected sibling pairs. *British Journal of Psychiatry*, **158**, 624–629.

[7] Coon H, Jensen S, Holik J *et al.* (1994). Genomic scan for genes predisposing to schizophrenia. *American Journal of Medical Genetics (Neuropsychiatric Genetics)*, **54**, 59–71.

[8] Schwab S G, Albus M, Hallmayer J (1995). Evaluation of a susceptibilty gene for schizophrenia on chromosome 6p by multipoint affected sib-pair linkage analysis. *Nature Genetics*, **11**, 325–327.

[9] Coon H, Sobell J, Heston L *et al.* (1994). Search for mutations in the β1 GABAa receptor subunit gene in patients with schizophrenia. *American Journal of Medical Genetics*, **54**, 12–20.

[10] Egeland J A, Gerhard D S *et al.* (1987). Bipolar affective disorder linked to DNA markers on Chromosome 11. *Nature*, **325**, 783–787.

[11] Hodgkinson S, Sherrington R, Gurling H *et al.* (1987). Molecular genetic evidence for heterogeneity in manic depression. *Nature*, **325**, 805–806.

[12] Robertson R (1987). Molecular Genetics of the mind. *Nature*, **325**, 755.

[13] Hardy J A, Higgins G A (1992). Alzheimer's disease: The amyloid cascade Alzheimer's Disease hypothesis. *Science*, **256**, 184–185.

[14] Su J H, Cummings B J, Cotman C W (1994). Early phosphorylation of tau in Alzheimer's disease occurs at ser-202 and is preferentially located within neurites. *Neuroreport*, **5**, 2358–2362.

[15] Smith M A, Siedlak S L, Richey P L *et al.* (1995). Tau protein interacts with the amyloid-β-protein: implications for Alzheimer's disease. *Nature Medicine*, **1**, 365–369.

[16] Goate A, Chartier-Harlin M, Mullan M *et al.* (1991). Segregation of a missense mutation in the amyloid precursor protein gene with familial Alzheimer's disease. *Nature*, **349**, 704–706.

[17] Hollands A J, Oliver C (1995). Down's syndrome and the links with Alzheimer's disease. *Journal of Neurology, Neurosurgery and Psychiatry*, **59**, 111–114.

[18] Pericak-Vance M, Bebout J, Gaskell P (1991). Linkage studies in familial Alzheimer's disease; evidence for chromosome 19 linkage. *American Journal of Human Genetics*, **48**, 1034–1050.

[19] Sherrington R, Rogaev E I, Liang Y *et al.* (1995). Cloning of a gene bearing missense mutations in early onset Alzheimer's disease. *Nature*, **375**, 754–760.

[20] Rogaev E I, Sherrington R, Rogaev E A *et al.* (1995). Familial Alzheimer disease kindreds with missense mutations on chromosome 1 related to the Alzheimer disease Type 3 gene. *Nature*, **375**, 754–760.

[21] Verkerk A J M H, Picretti M, Sutcliffe J S *et al.* (1991). Identification of a gene (FMR-1) containing a CGG repeat coincident with breakpoint cluster region exhibiting length variation in Fragile X syndrome. *Cell*, **65**, 905–914.

22 Huntington's Disease Collaborative Research Group (1993). A novel gene containing a trinucleotide repeat that is expanded and unstable on Huntington's disease chromosomes. *Cell*, **72**, 971–983.

23 Gortason R, Wahlstrom R (1991). Chromosomal alteration in the mildly mentally retarded. *Journal of Mental Deficiency*, 35, 240–246.

Chapter 9

Personality disorder

Chris Buller

Personality disorders are important to clinical practice and hence the MRCPsych examinations. Recent developments have focused on the understanding and treatment of the personality disorders, and also the impact of personality on Axis I disorders. It is important to note that:

- The concept of personality disorder lends itself well to essay questions.

- Most of the methodologically sound research has appeared in the last 5 years and as a result these topics are covered poorly in the major textbooks.

Chronological Development of the Concept

- **1801 – Pinel** used the term *"manie sans delire"* to describe individuals prone to unprovoked outbursts of rage and violence despite intact intellectual functions.[1]

- **1837 – J. C. Pritchard** wrote of *"moral insanity"*,

where the primary problem was a deficiency of morals, not of intellect.[2]

- **1889 – ICD 1**: *"moral and impulsive insanity"* became a diagnostic category.

- **1891 – Koch** introduced the term *"psychopathic"*.[3]

- **1923 – Schneider** produced an expanded classification of *"psychopathic personality disorder"*.[4] He was the first to emphasise that not only **society** but also the **sufferer** has to endure the consequences of personality abnormalities.

- **1936 – Kretschmer** used the term *"schizoid"*, describing individuals with the personality characteristics of paranoia, oversensitivity, shyness and suspiciousness.[5]

- **1941 – Cleckley's** book *The Mask of Sanity* suggested that psychopathy was the result of a pathological process.[6]

- **1958 – Chodoff and Lyons** describe a number of traits central to the concept of *"hysterical personality disorder"*.[7]

- **1960s and 1970s** – Dynamic theory and psychodynamic practice led to the concepts of *"narcissistic"* and *"borderline"* personality disorders.[8–10]

- **1980 – DSM-III** was the first International Classification containing diagnostic criteria for all categories including personality disorders.[11]

Current Classifications of Personality Disorders

- Both **ICD-10**[12] and **DSM-IV**[13] contain categories of personality disorder which differ only slightly in their nomenclature (Table 9.1), and both provide a brief description of each personality disorder type.[12, 13]

- DSM-IV contains diagnostic criteria for each personality disorder, whereas ICD-10 contains only guidelines.

- Since 1980, successive revisions of DSM have divided up the personality disorders into three loosely defined, and theoretically non-overlapping, clusters (Table 9.1). Much of the research that has been carried out in the United States refers to particular clusters of personality disorders rather than individual personality disorder types.

Table 9.1 Current classifications of personality disorder

Cluster	ICD-10	DSM-IV
A: (Odd/eccentric)	Paranoid	Paranoid
	Schizoid	Schizoid
	—[a]	Schizotypal
B: (Flamboyant/eccentric)	Histrionic	Histrionic
	Dyssocial	Dyssocial
	—[a]	Narcissistic
	Borderline	Borderline
	Impulsive	—[a]
C: (Fearful/anxious)	Anankastic	Anankastic
	Dependent	Dependent
	Anxious	Avoidant
	—[a]	Passive–aggressive

[a] No equivalent classification.

Epidemiology

Personality disorders are common. They have been identified in:

- 13% of urban adults.[14]

- 34% of patients with conspicuous psychiatric morbidity attending urban general practices,[15] and 20% of patients attending rural practices.[16]

- 34% of patients presenting as a psychiatric emergency to an inner London teaching hospital.[17]

- Nearly 50% of psychiatric in-patients.[18]

- 60% of parasuicides.[19]

- There is general agreement that personality disorders are more common in males and in urban populations and show a decreasing rate with increasing age. There is a possibility that this reflects the altered personality as a result of increased maturity or altered social circumstances (relationships, families, jobs, etc.) that may occur with age.

Treatment of Personality Disorders

Over the last decade there has been a steady increase in the amount of research into the treatment of these disorders, particularly in the United States. A major stimulus for research was the inclusion of diagnostic criteria in DSM-III for each personality disorder type. This allowed treatment trials to be carried out in well defined patient groups. As a result, a variety of biological and psychotherapeutic treatments have been suggested for both specific personality disorders and also symptom clusters which are common to more than one personality disorder type, such as impulsivity/aggressiveness.

Pharmacotherapy

Until the mid-1980s there were few methodologically sound drug studies, and those that did appear in the literature focused mainly on the pharmacotherapy of borderline personality disorder (see box). This was chiefly because borderline patients did not do well in psychoanalysis but frequently presented for treatment.

DSM-IV diagnostic criteria for borderline personality disorder

Five of the following nine criteria:

1. Frantic efforts to avoid real or imagined abandonment.

2. Unstable and intense inter-personal relationships.

3. Identity disturbance.

4. Impulsivity in at least two areas such as spending, sex, substance abuse, binge eating and reckless driving.

5. Recurrent suicidal behaviour.

6. Affective instability.

7. Chronic feelings of emptiness.

8. Inappropriate, intense anger or difficulties controlling anger.

9. Transient, stress-related paranoid ideation or severe dissociative symptoms.

The range of drugs that may be used to treat personality disorders include:

Low-dose neuroleptics

- Since the 1950s low-dose neuroleptics have been used by a number of American psychoanalysts to help borderline patients cope with the stresses and strains of therapy.

- Soloff *et al.*[20] conducted the first placebo-controlled trial of antipsychotic medication in borderline personality disorder (BPD) and schizotypal personality disorder (SPD) patients. Low doses of haloperidol (mean = 7.25 mg) were effective against a wide range of symptoms including depression, anxiety, hostility, paranoid ideation and psychoticism. However, the same group later found no difference between haloperidol and placebo in the treatment of borderline patients, except for subjective anger and behavioural dyscontrol.[21]

- Another group compared continuation treatment with haloperidol and phenelzine in patients with BPD, but came to the conclusion that *"there is currently no clear pharmacological treatment of choice for the continuation therapy of BPD"*.[22]

- It appears that in borderline and schizotypal patients the major tranquillisers have little more to offer than "tranquillisation".

Tricyclic antidepressants

- Early American studies were flawed by methodological problems. In the only methodologically sound treatment trial, Soloff *et al.*[20] found that the depressed borderline and schizotypal patients treated with amitriptyline (average daily dose = 148 mg) did only slightly better on the Beck and Hamilton rating scales than the depressed subjects on placebo.

- More recent work has concentrated on the effectiveness of tricyclics in the treatment of dysthymia. Marin *et al.*[23] conducted a prospective, non-blind, 8-week trial comparing the response rates of patients with dysthymia and double depression (defined as a depressive disorder supervening on longer term dysthymic personality). Treatment with desipramine (average daily dose = 221 mg) led to complete or partial remission in 70% of patients with dysthymia. However, there was no placebo comparison group and subjects were recruited for this study by newspaper advertisement.

Monoamine oxidase inhibitors (MAOIs)

- There have been a few reports in the literature of MAOIs being effective in the treatment of borderline personality disorder.

- In a small, longitudinal, crossover, placebo-controlled trial, Cowdrey and Gardner[24] found **tranylcypromine** produced an improvement in the symptoms of anxiety, depression and the sensitivity to rejection that are frequently seen in borderline patients.

- Soloff *et al*[22] also found **phenelzine** to be effective against a wide range of borderline symptoms.

Selective serotonin reuptake inhibitors (SSRIs)

- Fluoxetine has been found to be effective in a number of impulsive disorders such as obsessive–compulsive disorder and bulimia. It is not surprising then that researchers have investigated the efficacy of SSRIs in borderline personality disorder where impulsivity is a common feature.

- Markovitz *et al*.[25] reported a tenfold reduction in the rate of self-mutilation in 22 out-patients with BPD over a 12-week study period using **fluoxetine**. The limitations of the study included the small sample size, and lack of a clinical assessment scale or a control group.

- Kavoussi *et al*.[26] carried out an open 8-week trial of **sertraline** (dose range 50–200 mg) in a small number of predominantly BPD patients. The authors reported a significant reduction in the amount of overt aggression and irritability that was displayed by subjects who remained in the trial for at least 4 weeks.

- **SSRIs** have also been used in the treatment of **dysthymia**. Hellerstein *et al*.[27] conducted an 8-week double-blind study of fluoxetine versus placebo in the treatment of dysthymia in 35 out-patients. Only 19% of patients treated with placebo improved compared to 63% of fluoxetine-treated patients.

Mood stabilisers

- **Lithium** has been found to be effective in reducing the frequency of assaultative behaviour in seriously violent prison inmates.[28] However, for ethical reasons it is unlikely that this type of study will ever be repeated.

- A 6-week double-blind crossover trial[24] demonstrated the efficacy of **carbamazepine** in treating the behavioural dyscontrol that is frequently seen in borderline personality disorder patients. However, in this particular study the sample size was small ($n = 14$) and 4 out of 14 patients developed allergic skin reactions whilst on carbamazepine.

Psychotherapeutic approaches

Focused psychological treatments

- This strategy aims for some slight improvement, rather than long-term personality change and is **focused** (on particular problem areas) and **short-term** (10–20 weeks).

- Most psychological treatments of this type tend to be **behavioural** or **cognitive–behavioural** in approach.

- Most therapists **target specific symptom clusters**, e.g. anxiety in social situations, lack of confidence, problems with assertiveness, or anger.

- There has hitherto been a lack of methodologically sound studies supporting the efficacy of psychological treatments, although evidence is slowly growing.

Assessment should include a **behavioural analysis** aimed at identifying:

- **Precipitating factors**, e.g. rejection, an argument.

- **Associated emotions**, e.g. tension, anger, low mood.

- **Cognitions preceding problem behaviour**, e.g. self-harm may be associated with the thoughts such as *"I hate myself"*, *"I am worthless"*.

- **Associated behaviours**, e.g. the sociopath looking for a weapon, the self-harmer searching for medication to take as an overdose.

- **Factors increasing likelihood of problem behaviour**, e.g. alcohol, isolation.

- **Factors decreasing likelihood of problem behaviour**, e.g. strenuous exercise, contacting a confidante, using distraction techniques.

- **Listing the benefits**, e.g. reduction of tension, **and drawbacks**, e.g. guilt and self-loathing after the behaviour.

Treatment of impulsivity

Impulsivity is a common feature of a number of personality disorder types:

- Dyssocial personality disorder.

- Emotionally unstable personality disorder: impulsive and borderline types.

- Histrionic personality disorder.

It may manifest as repeated episodes of deliberate self-harm, aggression or binge eating or drinking.

One of the main aims of treatment is to disrupt the sequence of events that culminates in the impulsive behaviour. For example:

- **Cognitive techniques** can be applied to the low self-esteem that underlies dysfunctional assumptions that many of these patients hold, e.g. *"I'm worthless"* (see Chapter 5).

- **Behavioural techniques** aim at disrupting associated behaviours.

- Teaching the repetitive self-harmer effective **distraction techniques** (e.g. to seek out company, not isolation, when they are ruminating over self-harm).

- **Relaxation therapy** may be helpful in reducing the build-up of tension as may strenuous physical exercise. This may help them to cope more effectively with previously intolerable emotions.

- **Problem solving**. Teaching patients how to solve the problems that previously seemed to overwhelm them may be an effective intervention. Salkovskis *et al.*[29] showed that this reduces the risk of further overdose amongst recurrent deliberate self-harming patients. This may include new skills of coping such as assertiveness and social skills training (described below).

- Anger may be discharged by pummelling cushions or helped by the more formal approach of **anger management** (see below).

Anger management

- A behavioural approach is indicated for those prone to aggressive outbursts. This identifies antecedants (such as abuse of drink) that are associated with angry outbursts.

- The patient re-enacts some previous episode of aggressive behaviour and the therapist uses role-play, assertiveness training and distraction techniques to teach more appropriate responses.

- The patient learns to detect times when they are at risk of becoming angry, and discovers other ways of dealing more effectively with the situation.

Social skills and assertiveness training

- Useful for those individuals who are socially anxious, lacking in confidence and have problems with assertiveness.

- Often carried out as an **assertiveness course,** typically of 8–10 individuals in a group (although may be done individually). Uses education, role-play and feedback to teach new skills of assertiveness. Techniques include "broken record", etc.

Longer-term psychotherapeutic treatments aiming at personality change

Group psychotherapy

A therapeutic community (e.g. the Cassell Hospital) is probably the best treatment for dyssocial personality disorder. In this environment individuals start to understand what it is like to be on the receiving end of antisocial behaviour, and this encourages the taking of responsibility for one's behaviour. It draws upon the principles of a "**therapeutic community**", a term first used by **Main** in 1946.[30] **Rapoport**,[31] at the Henderson hospital, specified four key components:

- **Communalism** – equal shares for all.
- **Democratization** – abolition of hierarchy.
- **Permissiveness** – tolerance of disturbed behaviour.
- **Reality confrontation** – regular feedback to individuals of the results of their behaviour.

Individual psychotherapy

This has been advocated for patients with borderline, schizotypal, narcissistic and hysterical personality disorders. However, there has been little evaluation of this treatment method in these groups. In probably the best study to date, Mehlum *et al.*[32] followed up 97 personality-disordered patients who were treated at a specialist day unit. They received psychodynamic psychotherapy, both individually and in groups, within the framework of a therapeutic community. The authors found that at the end of a 3-year period:

- Patients with borderline personality disorder displayed a moderate symptom reduction and a fair global outcome.

- Patients with schizotypal personality disorder showed a similar reduction in symptoms but relatively poor global functioning.

- Patients with Cluster C personality disorders (anxious/avoidant, anankastic, and dependent types) showed both a good global outcome and marked symptom reduction.

Co-morbidity and Personality Disorders

Personality disorder and other (Axis I) mental illness can co-exist. Tyrer *et al.*[33] carried out a survey in the United Kingdom and identified a personality disorder in:

- 59% of patients with alcohol dependence.

- 55% of patients with schizophrenia.

- 40% of patients with manic depressive illness.

Co-morbidity with neuroses

Cluster C personality disorders have often been found to be associated with neurotic diagnoses such as panic disorder, agoraphobia and social phobia.[34]

Co-morbidity with depression

Shea *et al.*[35] reviewed the data on the prevalence of personality disorder in both depressed in-patients and out-patients. They noted that Cluster B personality disorders (histrionic, dyssocial, borderline and narcissistic types) are commoner in in-patient groups whereas Cluster C personality disorders are more frequent in depressed out-patients.

Co-morbidity with other disorders

- Eating disorders are commonly associated with personality disorders. Fahy *et al.*[36] found that **39%** of a sample of **bulimic** patients satisfied the diagnostic criteria for personality disorder (mainly anxious and histrionic types).

- Rost *et al.*[37] found **37%** of a sample of 94 **somatisers** also had a personality disorder (mainly avoidant, paranoid, self-defeating and anankastic types).

- Dyssocial personality disorder has been found in **44%** of **opiate abusers**.[38] Opiate abusers with co-morbid dyssocial personality disorder also had higher rates of HIV seropositivity than opiate abusers without this Axis II diagnosis.

Implications of co-morbidity for treatment

In recent years a number of studies have been published that have focused on the extent to which a patient's personality status may impede the response to treatment of a co-existent Axis I disorder. Recent studies have involved depressed patients in primary care, out-patients with neurotic disorders, patients with obsessive–compulsive disorder and bulimic out-patients (Table 9.2).

These studies appear to indicate that:

- Patients with both an Axis I disorder and an Axis 2 (personality) disorder tend to display **more severe symptomatology** when they are first referred for treatment than those patients without a personality disorder.

- Patients with either a neurotic or depressive illness plus a personality disorder **do** respond to psychotropic medication. However, the **therapeutic response appears to be delayed** in these patients compared with those who present solely with either a neurotic or depressive illness.

- It is **not always** the case that presence of a personality disorder indicates a poor outcome of a co-existent Axis I disorder.

Key points

Principles of management of personality disorders:

- **Always treat any co-existent Axis I disorder** (e.g. depressive episodes, panic attacks, alcohol and drug dependence).

- The aim of therapy should be **progress in specific areas of functioning**. Total change is over-optimistic and rarely possible.

- Remember **progress will be slow** and patients are better seen regularly for short periods, over a number of years than intensely over a few weeks.

- **Treatment goals should be clearly set out** before embarking on brief or focal psychotherapies.

- **Care must be taken when it comes to prescribing** for these patients. Beware of fostering drug dependency. Benzodiazepines are clearly contraindicated apart from their use in detoxification, and there is the risk of releasing self-harming behaviour as a result of behavioural disinhibition. Avoid, if possible, prescribing drugs that are toxic in overdose, e.g. tricyclics; choose if possible a safer preparation. Limit the supplies of drug, or make sure they are looked after by a relative, Community Psychiatric Nurse, etc.

Table 9.2 Outcome studies

Reference	Diagnostic group	Study type	Main findings
Baer et al.[39]	Obsessive compulsive disorder (OCD)	Prospective, non-blind, 12 week treatment trial of clomipramine 100–300 mg/day in 55 patients with OCD	1. 60% of sample met DSM-III-R criteria for personality disorder (PD). Most were Cluster C 2. Presence of a PD was not related to treatment outcome; however, patients with Cluster A PDs had more severe OCD symptoms initially and had a poorer outcome. Also, the presence of avoidant and borderline PDs, along with total number of PDs, predicted a poorer treatment outcome 3. Main weakness of this study was that patients were excluded if they possessed personality traits that may have interfered with compliance
Fahy et al.[36]	Bulimia nervosa	Prospective, non-blind, 8-week trial of cognitive-behaviour therapy in 39 female out-patients.	1. 39% of sample were identified as having a PD by the personality assessment schedule (PAS) 2. At the start of the trial bulimics with a PD were more depressed and weighed less than those without

Table 9.2 cont.,

		3. Presence of a PD was not related to a poorer treatment outcome; however, PD + bulimia + depression + low weight predicted a poorer response
Tyrer et al.[40]	Generalised anxiety disorder, panic disorder and dysthymia	Randomised placebo-controlled 10-week trial of CBT vs. self-help vs. drug treatment in 181 out-patients. Two-year follow-up
		1. Similar response of generalised anxiety disorder, panic disorder and dysthymia to all three types of treatment
		2. Patients without PD initially displayed less psychopathology and showed a better response to psychological treatments.
		3. Antidepressant treatment was more effective than psychological treatments in patients with PD
Patience et al.[41]	Depressive illness	Randomised 16-week trial comparing CBT, counselling, routine GP care and drug treatment by a psychiatrist in 113 depressed primary care patients
		1. 26% of sample were identified as having a personality disorder by the PAS
		2. Presence of a PD delays recovery from a major depressive episode but at 18-month follow-up no difference between PD and no PD groups

References

[1] Pinel P A (1801). *Treatise on Insanity* (trans. Davis DD, 1962). New York: Hafner.
[2] Pritchard J C (1837). *A Treatise on Insanity and Other Diseases Affecting the Mind.* Philadelphia: Harwell, Barrington and Harwell.
[3] Koch J L A (1891). *Die psychopathischen Minderwertigkeiten.* Dorn: Ravensberg.
[4] Schneider K. (1923). *Die Psychopathischen Personlichkeiten.* Berlin: Springer.
[5] Kretschmer E (1936). *Physique and Character,* 2nd edition (revised Miller). London: Routledge and Kegan Paul.
[6] Cleckley H (1941). *The Mask of Sanity.* London: Henry Kimpton.
[7] Chodoff P, Lyons H (1958). Hysteria: the hysterical personality and "hysterical conversion". *American Journal of Psychiatry,* **114**: 734.
[8] Kernberg O F (1975). *Borderline Conditions and Pathological Narcissism.* New York: Jason Aronson.
[9] Kohut H (1971). *The Analysis of the Self.* New York: International Universities Press.
[10] Gunderson J G, Singer M T (1975). Defining borderline patients: an overview. *American Journal of Psychiatry,* **132**, 1–10.
[11] *Diagnostic and Statistical Manual of Mental Disorders,* 3rd edition (1980). Washington, D.C.: American Psychiatric Association.
[12] *International Classification of Diseases and Related Health Problems* (ICD-10). (1993). Geneva: World Health Organization.
[13] *Diagnostic and Statistical Manual of Mental Disorders* (DSM-IV) (1993). Washington, D.C.: American Psychiatric Association.
[14] Casey P R, Tyrer P J (1986). Personality, functioning and symptomatology. *Journal of Psychiatric Research,* **20**, 363–374.
[15] Casey P R, Tyrer P J, Dillon S (1984). The diagnostic status of patients with conspicuous psychiatric morbidity in primary care. *Psychological Medicine,* **14**, 673–681.
[16] Casey P R (1985). Psychiatric morbidity in general practice: a diagnostic approach. MD thesis, National University of Ireland.
[17] Tyrer P, Merson S, Onyett S, Johnson T (1994). The effect of personality disorder on clinical outcome, social networks and adjustment: a controlled clinical trial of psychiatric emergencies. *Psychological Medicine,* **24**(3), 731–740.
[18] Dahl A. (1986). Some aspects of the DSM-III personality disorders illustrated by a consecutive series of hospitalised patients. *Acta Psychiatrica Scandinavica,* **73**, 61–66.
[19] Casey P R (1989). Suicide intent and personality disorder. *Acta Psychiatrica Scandinavica,* **79**, 290–295.
[20] Soloff P H, George A, Nathan R S et al. (1986). Progress in pharmacotherapy of borderline disorders: a double blind study of amitriptyline, haloperidol and placebo. *Archive of General Psychiatry,* **43**, 691–697.
[21] Soloff P H, Cornelius J, George A et al. (1993). Efficacy of phenelzine and

haloperidol in borderline personality disorder. *Archive of General Psychiatry,* **50,** 377–385.

[22] Cornelius J, Soloff P H, Perel J M, Uhlrich R F (1993). Continuation pharmacotherapy of borderline personality disorder with haloperidol and phenelzine. *American Journal of Psychiatry,* **150,** 1843–1848.

[23] Marin D B, Kocsis J H, Francos A J, Parides M (1994). Desipramine in the treatment of "pure" dysthymia vs. double depression. *American Journal of Psychiatry,* **151,** 1079–1080.

[24] Cowdrey R W, Gardner D L (1988). Pharmacotherapy of borderline personality disorder: alprazolam, carbamazepine, trifluoperazine and tranylcypromine. *Archives of General Psychiatry,* **45,** 111–119.

[25] Markovitz P J, Calabrese J R, Schulz S C, Meltzer H Y (1991). Fluoxetine in the treatment of borderline and schizotypal personality disorder. *American Journal of Psychiatry,* **148,** 1064–1067.

[26] Kavoussi R J, Liu J, Caccaro E F (1994). An open trial of sertraline in personality disordered patients with impulsive aggression. *Journal of Clinical Psychiatry,* **55:** 137–141.

[27] Hellerstein D J, Yanowitch P, Rosenthal J *et al.* (1993). A randomised double-blind study of fluoxetine versus placebo in the treatment of dysthymia. *American Journal of Psychiatry,* **150,** 1169–1175.

[28] Sheard M H, Marini J L, Bridges C I *et al.* (1976). The effect of lithium on unipolar aggressive behaviour in man. *American Journal of Psychiatry,* **133,** 1409–1413.

[29] Salkovskis P M, Atha C, Storer D (1990). Cognitive-behavioural problem-solving in the treatment of patients who repeatedly attempt suicide. A controlled trial. *British Journal of Psychiatry,* **157,** 871–876.

[30] Main T F (1946). The hospital as a therapeutic institution. *Bulletin of the Menninger Clinic,* **10,** 66–70.

[31] Rapoport R N (1960). *Community as Doctor: New Perspectives on a Therapeutic Community.* London: Tavistock Publications.

[32] Mehlum L, Friis S, Irion T *et al.* (1991). Personality disorders 2–5 years after treatment: a prospective follow-up study. *Acta Psychiatrica Scandinavica,* **84,** 72–77.

[33] Tyrer P, Casey P, Ferguson B (1988). Personality disorder and mental illness. In *Personality Disorders: diagnosis, management and course,* (ed.) P. Tyrer. London: Wright, pp. 93–104.

[34] Brown T A, Barlow D H (1992). Comorbidity among anxiety disorders: implications for treatment and DSM-IV. *Journal of Consulting and Clinical Psychology,* **60,** 835–844.

[35] Shea M T, Widiger T A, Klein M H (1992). Comorbidity of personality disorder and depression: Implications for treatment. *Journal of Consulting and Clinical Psychology,* **60,** 857–868.

[36] Fahy T A, Eisler I, Russell G F M (1993). Personality disorder and treatment response in Bulimia Nervosa. *British Journal of Psychiatry,* **162,** 765–770.

[37] Rost K M, Akins R N, Brown F W, Smith G R (1992). The comorbidity of DSM-III-R personality disorders in Somatisation Disorder. *General and Hospital Psychiatry,* **14,** 1241–1243.

[38] Brooner R K, Greenfield L, Schmidt C W, Bigelow G E (1993). Antisocial personality disorder and HIV infection among intravenous drug abusers. *American Journal of Psychiatry*, **150**, 53–58.

[39] Baer L, Jenike M A, Black W *et al.* (1992). Effect of Axis II diagnoses on treatment outcome with clomipramine in 55 patients with obsessive-compulsive disorder. *Archives of General Psychiatry*, **49**, 862–866.

[40] Tyrer P, Seivewright N, Ferguson B *et al.* (1993). The Nottingham study of neurotic disorder: effect of personality status on response to drug treatment, cognitive therapy and self-help over two years. *British Journal of Psychiatry*, **162**, 219–226.

[41] Patience D A, McGuire R J, Scott A I F, Freeman C P L (1995). The Edinburgh primary care depression study: personality disorder and outcome. *British Journal of Psychiatry*, **167**, 324–330.

Chapter 10

Community care

Asma Humayun

For two centuries the care of mentally ill people was largely isolated behind what are now thought of as the "forbidding gates" of the asylums. This is somewhat ironic since the advent of the asylums (providing a place of sanctuary) was initially a major advance in the humane care of the mentally ill. They relieved the community of the burden of patient care; nursing, protecting and ensuring the survival of the mentally ill.

Over the latter part of this century in particular, changes in social ideology have placed mental hospitals under tremendous pressure. Ongoing criticism, together with financial and other pressures, has moved the focus of care back to the concept of community-based services. In spite of the enthusiasm behind this concept, care in the community has taken over 30 years to establish and still has to fully prove its place as an effective approach to the care of the mentally ill. An urgent re-evaluation of the mental health-care system is necessary, to ensure suitable care of the mentally ill.

Asylums – an Historical Review

The decline in popularity of mental hospitals, and the growing scandal of sub-standard care provided in these institutions, started in the 1930s. A number of factors contributed towards this enormous change:

1. **Treatment innovations**:
   The introduction of pharmacological treatments, like **phenothiazines in 1957**, is believed to have profoundly influenced the role of the institutions. The bed occupancy in both the United Kingdom and the United States peaked in the mid 1950s, and has consistently fallen subsequently. Attributing the down turn of bed occupancy entirely to the advent of effective anti-psychotic medication is an oversimplification, particularly since the rates began to fall in the early 1950s.[1]

2. **Disenchantment with the mental hospitals**:
   The growing concern was that the mental hospitals were prolonging and adding to the disabilities caused by mental disorders. The most influential work came from **Irving Goffman** (*Asylums*)[2] who criticised the pathological features of institutions and introduced the concept of **Total Institutions** characterised by:

   - **Batch living**: described as the antithesis of domestic living: in institutional living the three spheres of home, work and play are collapsed into one.

   - **Binary management**: means that staff and inmates live in different worlds. Staff tend to feel "superior and righteous", while inmates are made to feel "weak, inferior and guilty".

   - **Inmate role**: this role is taught starting with a highly ritualised admissions procedure to **shape and code** the person into the patient role.

   - **Institutional perspective**: a view of life which validates the institution's existence to create an artificial sense of community and deny individual experiences.

Russell Barton[3] suggested that the "defect state" in chronic schizophrenia was **caused** by the mental hospitals.

3. **Conceptual developments**:
    In the 1960s the mental hospitals came under increasing pressure by a series of scandals, revealing cruel and degrading treatments in long-stay mental hospitals. The **anti-psychiatry** movement (e.g. **Thomas Szasz,**[4] **R D Laing**[5]) challenged the validity and utility of psychiatric diagnosis. At the same time, publicity surrounding treatments such as psychosurgery and electroconvulsive therapy added to the society's distaste for the then standard practice.

4. **Social policy changes**:
    The policy of **deinstitutionalisation** continued, and the change in the Government's approach was highlighted by the Member of Parliament **Enoch Powell**'s much-noted speech in 1961, when he foresaw the "demolition of brooding mental hospitals and their replacement by modern and acceptable services".

5. **Research findings**:
    Wing and Brown[6] illustrated that an under-stimulating environment might actually be harmful by contributing to the social handicaps of the chronic patients. Their well-known **three hospitals study** compared the outcome results of three different hospitals which had very different styles of patient care.

International developments

The developments in the United Kingdom (e.g. incorporation of mental health services into the **National Health Service** (1948) and **Mental Health Act** (1959)), emphasised the integration of social and health provision. These were paralleled with similar changes in the rest of Europe and the United States:

- The American **Community Mental Health Centre** movement launched by President J. Kennedy arrived at similar policy changes.
- **Italian Reforms – Law 180 (1978)** – stimulated a massive shift of emphasis in mental health care in the north of Italy. The radical decision to **completely close** all asylums has led to a mixed outcome and has been highly controversial.

The Concept of Community Care

The first official use of the term **community care** was in the **Annual Report of the Board of Control** (of mental hospitals) in **1930**. The concept developed with the decline of the mental hospital population, and has recently gained further momentum. The term is imprecise, however, and controversial.

- The term **community** has no defining boundaries and tends to be taken as "everything except the hospital".

- The process of **deinstitutionalisation** means "leaving the hospital", for care in the "community". The provision of care in the community has not progressed as fast as the move to discharge patients, and therefore some patients experience significant difficulties when they leave hospital.

- The exact number of hospital beds for people with long-term mental illness is not known. The hospital closure program began in 1954, when the number of psychiatric beds peaked at 148 000, and it aimed at reducing beds to a target of 47 900.

- By 1990, 64 000 remained.[7, 8] The Government document, *Caring for People*[9] (based on the work of Sir Roy Griffiths) implied that there is a wide range of voluntary services for people with mental illness, and that one key to effective care is the organisation and mobilisation of these resources. Provision in the private sector is certainly growing, and can be very effective, yet care is still patchily distributed.

- There is evidence that many of those discharged have been lost to follow-up. Nearly 100 000 long-stay patients have been discharged from British mental hospitals in the last 35 years, yet only 4000 places had been provided in local authority hostels by 1990.[8]

- There has been an increase in the number of cases of mental illness in the prison system that seems to have paralleled the number of patients discharged from the asylums.

There is clearly still a need for asylums with a range of acute and chronic wards. Young people with relapsing psychotic illnesses and disabilities have been left behind in the move to the community setting. They now make up the **new long-stay** population. Much has been written about this population, particularly in a series of studies by **Robin McCreadie** that have appeared regularly in the *British Journal of Psychiatry* over the past few years. The patients that seem to be losing out in the allocation of community resources are those with chronic psychiatric difficulties. This group create a **revolving door** effect, being admitted and re-admitted again and again, sometimes for short periods of time. This may partly be due to self-discharge or a refusal to take medication such as depots. One study looking at patients admitted seven or more times to a psychiatric hospital within a 2-year period found that only 2% of patients accounted for over 7% of all in-patients bed use in a general psychiatric unit:[10]

- Community care seems to work best for those with a mild degree of disability, good communication skills, an active social network and stable and predictable behaviour. In practice, however, community resources such as day hospitals and community psychiatric clinics may be used up by those who are not suffering from serious mental disorder, and yet demand help. In practice, this may include those with personality difficulties and those with milder psychiatric disorders.

- Community care is also reasonably successful for people with learning disability, the infirm elderly and physically handicapped, where the effective targeting of community resources such as Community Psychiatric Nurses, District Nurses and the use of day hospitals may be very effective.

Evaluation and follow-up studies of discharged long-stay patients

The traditional functions of mental hospitals have not and cannot be totally replicated in the community. Treatment of patients in the community is certainly possible, and the emphasis has been on **rehabilitation**, developing **after-care programmes**, and shifting the resources towards services in the community (**reprovision**). A number of approaches have been studied.

The Team for the Assessment of Psychiatric Services (TAPS) Project[11] is the most carefully researched reprovision exercise in the United Kingdom. Using cohorts of "leavers" and "stayers", the progress of 278 chronic patients with serious mental illness in Friern, Barnet and Claybury Hospitals has been studied. Those who were discharged into the community after extensive stays in hospital (movers), were meticulously monitored and compared with matched patients who remained in hospital (stayers). Most patients had schizophrenia. While a substantial proportion were re-admitted for brief periods, very few were lost to follow-up or became homeless. Patients demonstrated a **modest increase in**

their level of social interaction and a **marked improvement in satisfaction** with their lives and treatment. At 1-year follow-up, movers and stayers had the same death rate. Movers showed no significant improvement in psychiatric symptoms, but preferred their accommodation and the ability to be able to choose what to do with their time. The costs were about 10% less than that of in-patient care.[12] After 2 years there was also a suggestion of improvement in aspects of their clinical functioning.

Alternatives to hospitalisation studies

There are a number of well conducted studies offering patients community support as an alternative to hospital admission (reviewed by Braun *et al.*[13]). Important problems with these studies include:

- **Charismatic leaders** (product champions) who enthusiastically ensure that the approach works. Thus findings cannot easily be generalised to other settings.

- Studies examining only the **early stages of practice**.

- **Hawthorn effect** of a major study (i.e. the very action of offering any intervention creates a therapeutic impact).

- Enhanced or **better resourced** or informed clinical teams and **restricted entry** of patients which skew the results.

- **Poor quality control groups**.

Despite these reservations, there is accumulating evidence in favour of community psychiatry. The most influential studies are:

- **Stein and Test (1980).**[14] This study carried out in Australia demonstrated clinical, social and financial benefits, but also showed that withdrawal of the special team led to loss of all the gains. They introduced the importance of **assertive outreach** – the need to actively seek out those patients who default from treatment.

- **Dean and Gadd (1990).**[15] This is a study of **intensive home treatment (IHT)** for acute mental illness. Again benefits were found in social, clinical, financial and satisfaction ratings. Drawbacks of this study are a very special catchment area and the demands on the clinical teams.

- **Muijen** *et al.* **(1992).**[16, 17] This replicated the Stein and Test study at the Maudsley Hospital and confirmed the same findings.

Criticism of the Concept of Community Care

Community care has been exposed to large amounts of press coverage and public criticism in the last few years. The scandals were highlighted and dramatised where the services seemed inadequate to provide effective care of the mentally ill in the community.

- **Sensational headlines** like *"One murder a fortnight by mentally ill"* (*Daily Telegraph*), called for immediate action after 34 murders by the mentally ill over 18 months. Many were recently discharged and had recent contact with the psychiatric services prior to the incidents.

- An **inquiry** was held following the killing of 11-year-old **Emma Broadie** at Doncaster shopping centre in 1991 by **Carol Barratt**, who was discharged from a Section two days before the tragedy.

- A case which highlighted similar failings to act on warning signs was that of **Christopher Clunis**, a schizophrenic who stabbed and killed a complete stranger, **Jonathan Zito**, at a London underground station.

- **Ben Silcock** was mauled by a lion at London Zoo.

- The care worker **Jonathon Newby** was killed by a patient, **Jonathon Rous**.

These various factors have contributed to a growing concern regarding the safety of the mentally ill in the community, within the setting of continued political debate about inadequate funding for community care. The political outcome was a demand for changes in care by the Department of Health.

Efforts to Improve Care in the Community

1. In response to mounting criticism during the 1980s, the Government produced a White Paper entitled *Caring for People: Community Care in the Next Decade and Beyond.*[9] There has been further legislation in the **NHS and Community Care Act** (1990). Local authorities are now required to produce and publish community care plans for their area, to provide assessments of people likely to require community care services, and to set up care management systems.

2. **The care programme approach (CPA)** had its origins in the Spokes Inquiry into the care and aftercare of Sharon Campbell.[18] Its recommendations led to the publcication of a document by the Royal College of Psychiatrists.[19] This document provides a framework for good practice in delivering care to people

accepted by psychiatric services. CPA involves:

- Assessment of health and social care needs.
- A key worker to co-ordinate care.
- A written care plan.
- Regular review.
- Interprofessional collaboration.
- Consultation with users and carers.

In practice, the care programme approach tends to be formally applied in the following three situations:

- Patients discharged from hospital after being detained under Section 2, 3 or 37 of the Mental Health Act (1983).
- Patients who are discharged after being in hospital for 6 months or more.
- Patients who have complex needs requiring multi-disciplinary management. Collaboration and regular review will be facilitated by a formal care programme.

3. A **community supervision order** was proposed by the Royal College of Psychiatrists to ensure that "at-risk" patients maintain their treatment outside hospital and would permit early compulsory readmission to re-establish treatment if necessary. This was rejected by the Government after objections from pressure groups such as MIND on the basis of whether such an approach would infringe the rights of patients to refuse treatment. It was argued that such statutory powers might encourage lazy clinical practice, create an overemphasis on drugs, increase ethnic discrimination, and create problems with consent similar to those with Section 7 (guardianship) orders.[20]

4. Other possibilities to enhance care in the community included:

- **Supervised discharge**.

- **Extended leave of absence**.

- **Guardianship**.

The **Clunis inquiry** recommended special supervision to monitor **high risk** groups. The criteria proposed that certain patients be closely monitored:

- Those detained several times under the Mental Health Act.

- Those with a history of violence and persistent offending.

- Those failing to respond to treatment.

- The homeless.

5. The then Secretary of Health, **Virginia Bottomley**, put forward a **ten-point plan** and introduced **supervision registers**. She identified the patients who would fulfil criteria for inclusion on the register as those with **severe mental illness (including severe personality disorder** and **psychopathic disorder**) who are considered to be at significant risk of either **suicide** or **serious violence to others** or **severe self-neglect**.

There was some overlap between the recommendations of the Clunis inquiry and supervision registers, but the Health Secretary stressed that the focus must be on the most severely mentally ill – an estimated total of 8000 such patients in England and Wales.

The dilemma for the psychiatrist. The Royal College of Psychiatrists responded to the above proposals with some clear reservations:

- The criteria for inclusion are too broad. In Nottingham alone some 2000 such cases could be identified.

- Particularly in view of the inclusion of personality disorder, resources could be diverted away from those with severe mental illnesses.

- The estimated cost to implement the supervision register is approximately £77 million – although no extra funding was being made available by the Government.

- Clinically, it may be difficult to assess and, especially, to predict risk.

- It brings with it the risk of litigation and legal accountability for clinicians for the adequacy of follow-up and the action and safety of patients.

- Interference with the therapeutic relationship may occur as a result.

- Issues of confidentiality are raised, particularly as the team approach suggested may involve a range of professional and non-professional workers.

- Increasing paperwork and administration makes the procedure expensive in time and resources.[21,22]

Similar difficulties facing the psychiatrists were highlighted by Jeremy Coid in a *British Medical Journal* Editorial,[23] specifically that there are:

- No new legislative powers to enforce treatment if it is refused.

- No new resources.

- No guidance on level of professional accountability in future failures.

What of the Future?

- The current debate will continue to be a balance between offering appropriate patient care within a setting of limited financial resource.

- The right to be treated when ill and the right to reject admission or drug treatments for mental illness will remain a central issue.

Some proposed suggestions are:

- A lot more information is required to critically evaluate the whole concept of community care. There is an urgent need to collect data/facts. What is happening to patients who are discharged? Do the procedures that are currently offered work? If not, can they be improved?

- To clarify where the responsibility lies. The principle of **collective responsibility** (mental health teams) may be comforting to the team and protective from litigation, but does it help the patient not to know who is making the decisions?

- There are currently dangers with the introduction of new control systems (e.g. **community treatment orders**). Mental health legislation tends to be revised in a major way every 25 years, but it is currently only 12 years since the last significant revision. Considering the massive shift in provision of mental health services from the hospital to the "community", some feel that there is an urgent need for fundamental reform of current mental health legislation. Existing laws were designed when acute service provision was much more clearly in-patient based, it is perhaps unrealistic to expect them to work in the new system, with only the minor changes so far proposed.

Conclusions

Treatment has been transferred to the community but the traditional function of custodial care has not. The need to protect some people from their own actions when ill, and to protect the public from others, will always be there. "Special hospitals" and prisons are facing increasing demands, and it is likely that the community care debate will continue for many years.

Key points

- An understanding of the social, political and medical factors contributing to the shutdown of the asylums is essential.

- Research is needed to identify areas of need in the provision of community care.

- The identification of high risk or vulnerable patient groups has led to the development of innovative approaches to care.

- Difficulties for clinicians occur in implementing these proposals within a setting of limited financial resources. Good community care is possible, although expensive in terms of time and resources.

- Longer term changes in mental health legislation are needed which balance the rights of the individual to reject treatment against the right to be treated when ill and the right of others to live safely in the community.

- The community care approach will continue to

need to be supplemented by adequate in-patient facilities.

- The whole arena of community care issues will remain controversial and may remain dogged by the danger of adverse publicity.

References

[1] Warner R (1985). *Recovery from Schizophrenia: Psychiatry and Political Economy*. New York: Routledge and Kegan.

[2] Goffman E (1961). *Asylums: Essays on the Social Situation of Mental Patients and Other Inmates*. New York: Doubleday.

[3] Barton R (1965). *Institutional Neurosis*, 2nd edition. Southampton: Wiley.

[4] Szasz T (1963). *Law Liberty and Psychiatry*. New York: Macmillan.

[5] Laing R D (1960). *The Divided Self*, London: Tavistock.

[6] Wing J K, Brown G W (1961). Social treatment of chronic schizophrenia: A comparative survey of three mental hospitals. *Journal of Mental Science*, **107**, 847–861.

[7] Thornicroft G, Bebbington P (1990). Deinstitutionalisation: from hospital closure to service development. *British Journal of Psychiatry*, **155**, 739–753.

[8] Groves T (1990). After the asylums. What does community care mean now? *British Medical Journal*, **300**, 1060–1062.

[9] Secretaries of State for Health, Social Security, Wales and Scotland. (1989). *Caring for People: Community Care in the Next Decade and Beyond*. London: HMSO.

[10] Williams C J, Gilbody S, Kirby P (1996). Heavy psychiatric service users and the community care programme. Presented at the Annual Meeting of the Royal College of Psychiatrists, London, July 1996.

[11] Leff J, Thornicroft G (1993). TAPS project. *British Journal of Psychiatry*, **162**, Supplement 19.

[12] Marks I (1992). Innovations in mental health care delivery. *British Journal of Psychiatry*, **160**, 589–597.

[13] Braun P, Kochansky G, Shapiro R *et al.* (1981). Overview: deinstitutionalisation of psychiatric patients, a critical review of outcome studies. *American Journal of Psychiatry*, **138**(6), 736–749.

[14] Stein L I, Test M A. (1980). Alternative to mental hospital treatment. *Archives of General Psychiatry*, **37**, 392–397.

[15] Dean C, Gadd E M (1990). Home treatment for acute psychiatric illness. *British Medical Journal*, **301**, 1021–1023.

[16] Muijen M, Marks I M, Connolly J *et al.* (1992a). The daily living programme: preliminary comparison of community versus hospital based treatment for the

seriously mentally ill facing emergency admission. *British Journal of Psychiatry*, **160**, 379–384.

[17] Muijen M, Marks I M, Connolly J *et al*. (1992). Home based care and standard hospital care for patients with severe mental illness: A randomised controlled trial. *British Medical Journal*, **304**, 749–754.

[18] Department of Health and Social Security (1988). *Report of the Committee of Inquiry into the Care and Aftercare of Sharon Campbell (Chairman: J Spokes)*. London: HMSO.

[19] *Good Medical Practice in the Aftercare of Potentially Violent or Vulnerable Patients Discharged from In-patient Psychiatric Treatment* (1991). London: Royal College of Psychiatrists.

[20] Bluglass R (1993). New powers of supervised discharge of mentally ill people. *British Medical Journal*, **307**, 1160.

[21] Caldicott F (1994). Supervision registers: the College's response. *Psychiatric Bulletin*, **18**, 385–388.

[22] Guidance on the Introduction of Supervision Registers. (1994) London: Royal College of Psychiatrists.

[23] Coid J (1994). Failure in community care: psychiatry's dilemma. *British Medical Journal*, **308**, 805.

Chapter 11

Issues in transcultural psychiatry

Christine M. Hodgson-Nwaefulu

The purpose of this chapter is to give an overview of the key issues in transcultural psychiatry. Transcultural psychiatry has flourished over the past two decades. It incorporates a diverse range of disciplines, including psychiatry, sociology, medical anthropology, politics and economics. It is recognised to be important for the establishment of comprehensive mental health services, and for the training of health care workers.[1] In line with this stated importance, there is now a **Transcultural Special Interest Group** within the Royal College of Psychiatrists. The main emphasis in this chapter, as in much of the literature, is on black ethnic minority groups. It is important, however, to remember white ethnic minorities (e.g. East Europeans and Irish), who can also experience many similar difficulties.

Definitions (see Table 11.1)[2]

- **Race** is a classification of people based on visual observations, particularly skin colour. It is a biological myth, but continues to be a social reality. The genetic diversity **within** a "race" is greater than that between different "races".

- **Culture** is the non-physical influence on individuals that determines their behaviour, attitudes and ways of life; a "blue-print" for living. Culture is dynamic.

- **Ethnicity** implies a sense of **belonging**. Increasingly it is used to convey both a sense of cultural and social identity, without implying anything derogatory.

- **Ethnic minority** refers to a group of individuals who consider themselves separate from the general population, and are seen by the population at large to be distinct because of one or more of the following: common geographical or racial origin, skin colour, language, religious beliefs and practices, or dietary customs.[3] Ethnic minority groups are heterogeneous.

Table 11.1 Comparison of race, culture and ethnicity[2]

	Characterised by	Determined by	Perceived as
Race	Physical	Genetic	Permanent
Culture	Behaviour Attitudes	Upbringing Choice	Changeable Assimilation occurs
Ethnicity	Sense of belonging Group identity	Social pressure Psychological need	Situational/ negotiated Partially changeable

Other conceptual issues

- **Category fallacy**: refers to the assumption that Western diagnostic categories are themselves culture free entities; they are explanatory models specific to the Western context (e.g. International Pilot Study of Schizophrenia[4]). Culture does more than shape illness as an experience; it shapes the way we conceive of illness.[5]

- **Ethnocentricism**: assuming that everyone thinks and behaves the way oneself does, or stereotyping, attributing the same characteristics to all those in one group.

Models of Health and Illness

A culture provides guidelines for how to be acceptably deviant within a recognised pattern. There may be a great difference between the perceptions of professionals and those of service users in a multi-ethnic society. There may be differences in views of what constitutes illness, what causes illness, where it is appropriate to seek help, and what help is expected[6] (see Tables 11.2 and 11.3)

Table 11.2 Different understandings of mental health[7]

Eastern world view	Western world view
Integration and harmony:	Self-sufficiency
between person and environment	Assertiveness
between families	Competition
within societies	
in relation to spiritual values	
Social integration	Personal autonomy, independence
Balanced functioning	Efficiency
Protection and caring	Self-esteem
Self fulfilment dependent on:	
"Being"	"Doing"[8]
Communication emphasis on:	
Non-verbal	Verbal[8]

Table 11.3 Focus of intervention for mental health promotion[7]

Eastern	Western
Acceptance	Control
Harmony	Personal autonomy
Understanding by awareness	Understanding by analysis
Contemplation	Problem-solving
Body–mind–spirit unity	Body–mind separate (**Cartesian duality**)

Transcultural Approaches to Illness Presentation

Lexicon of affect (language of emotion)

- Some languages **do not have** verbal equivalents of "anxiety", "depression", etc.

- Western cultures tend to focus on **subjective feeling** component.[9]

The concept of **somatisation** may be useful in assessing the presentation of symptoms:

- **Somatisation** is "*a tendency to experience and communicate somatic distress and symptoms unaccounted for by pathological findings, to attribute them to physical illness, and to seek medical help for them*".[10]

- Or, in its broadest sense, somatisation is "*the expression of personal and social distress in an idiom of bodily complaints and medical help-seeking*".[11]

- Somatic symptoms in depression and anxiety play **a more central role** in the experience and expression of disorder in non-Western societies, and among ethnic minority groups in the West.[12]

- Somatic symptoms and **somatic metaphor** are, to some extent, used to communicate emotional distress in all cultures.[13]

- Differences in the conceptualisation of illness between western Europe and the "third world" results from the influence of biomedicine in association with industrialisation. It does **not** imply progression to more advanced "scientific" models.[14]

Detecting psychiatric disorders

Considering transcultural issues, **screening questionnaires** and **diagnostic instruments** need to:

- Be **conceptually valid** in each culture of use.

- Be comprehensive for the common somatic symptoms found **in each ethnic group**.

- Take account of **models of traditional healers** and folk categories of illness.

The **Bradford somatic inventory**[15] is a 21-item screening questionnaire. It aids identification of psychiatric disorders in Asian patients who present with somatic symptoms. A score greater than 14 implies 60% likelihood of a psychiatric disorder. The particular type of psychiatric disorder (anxiety state, depressive illness, etc.) needs to be established by further interview, preferably in the patient's first language.

Beliefs about traditional healers and the use of complementary therapies

- May be relevant in all patient groups.

- Often not readily admitted by the patient, fearing it to be unacceptable to the doctor.

- Knowledge of all therapies a patient is receiving is important in assessment.

- Many complementary therapies may be very helpful.

- A few have dangers or may interact.

- Compliance compromised if advice conflicts with that of traditional healer.[6]

Culture bound syndrome

This refers to disorders **restricted to a particular culture**, and resulting from a specific socio-cultural conflict or mode of thinking.[16] Examples include:

- Koro in South East Asia.

- Possession states in many cultures.

- Eating disorders in Western societies.

(Detailed examples are given elsewhere including Cox and Jorsh.[17])

Some feel that "culture bound syndrome" is a **redundant term**, as all reactions are, to an extent, culturally determined.[14]

Transcultural Factors in the Causation of Mental Illness

- **Migration.**[18] Mental illness may reflect:

  (i)   Pattern of disorder as in country of origin.

  (ii) Selection theory; more likely to migrate if have poor relationships, which may be due to the early stages of schizophrenia/other mental illness.

  (iii) Stress associated with migration and resettlement.

  (iv) Social isolation and insecurity, leading to paranoid ideation.

  (v)   Factors in the country of settlement.

- **Social class**: ethnic minorities in Britain, especially black people, are socially and economically disadvantaged; they face more obstacles in education, employment and promotion.[19]

- **Racism**: this has been socially constructed over hundreds of years and is a unique cause of stress for ethnic minorities. It also may create barriers to service access. It is present in systems of education, advertising, propaganda, political manipulations, economic pressure, and the ordinary "common sense" of the person in the street. It affects our perceptions of culture, and these assumptions are incorporated into the training of professionals.[7] Racism is a fact of life for black and ethnic minority people in Britain, occurring on both a personal and an institutional level.

The impact of migration

Migration is defined as *"the more or less permanent movement of persons or groups over a significant distance"*.[20] Regarding the United Kingdom, who came and when?

- Sizeable isolated minority communities have been established for generations in the United Kingdom (e.g. Bradford Asian population, Liverpool black population).[6]

- The most intense period of immigration of black people was during the economic boom in the 1950s and 1960s.

- Details on the migration of specific groups are described in detail by Rack[21] and Mares *et al*.[6]

Reasons for migration

- **Push factors**: poverty, high unemployment, lack of opportunity.
- **Pull factors**: acute labour shortage in Britain in

1950s and 1960s.

Difficulties caused by migration

- Split families (separation from rest of family for prolonged period).

- Loss of usual social and family support networks.

- Immigration restriction – waiting and uncertainty before being joined by family.

- Fears of deportation.

- Racism.

- Stress of living in a very different culture.

- Communication barriers: language, non-verbal communication, meanings.

- Isolation.

- Change of status: in family and employment.

- Lack of recognition of professional qualifications.

- Unemployment and poor housing.

- **Culture shock** : a feeling of **profound disorientation** experienced by an individual when plunged, with inadequate preparation, into an alien and potentially threatening culture.[22]

Stages of adjustment to migration (see Table 11.4)

Table 11.4 Adjustment possibilities[23]

		New culture valued	
		Yes	No
Old culture	**Yes**	Integration	Separation
valued	**No**	Assimilation	Marginalisation

- **Pre-immigration**: motivation for change needed.

- **Coping stage of immigration**:
  - (i) **Impact level** – elation, relief and fulfilment on arrival in the new country.
  - (ii) **Rebound level** – disappointment; anger or depression.
  - (iii) **Coping level** – learning and mastery of the new environment.

- **Settlement**: identifying with surroundings and developing sense of belonging.

- **Reverse culture shock** can occur on return to original country.[20]

- A greater chance of coping comes with **greater cohesion** within the immigrant group.

- There is a **need to grieve** for loss of the old culture, and resolve threat to one's own identity.

Epidemiology in Transcultural Psychiatry

Problems in cross-cultural epidemiological studies

1. **Misdiagnosis**:
   - **Diagnostic instruments** developed and standardized in the West may not be valid in other cultures. Most are based on psychological symptoms.

   - **Cultural pitfalls in diagnosis** of specific mental conditions are discussed in detail by Rack.[21] Understanding the social and cultural background of patients from ethnic minorities, and therefore the context in which psychiatric illness has occurred, is the key to a successful diagnosis.

2. **Inaccurate denominator**: no nationally collected reliable data on ethnic minority population size were gathered until the 1991 Census. This makes the accurate calculation of incidence, prevalence and relative risk of developing psychiatric illness fraught with difficulty.

3. **Experience of racism**:[24] this may affect both access to care, and also the quality of service offered.

4. **Differences in service use**: difficulties in access to services and stigma may lead to later presentation.

5. **Non-homogenous** nature of racial and ethnic groups. People are individuals and have their own very different personal needs.

6. **Confounding factors**, e.g. social class and unemployment.

Morbidity rates

Thomas *et al.*[25] note that several studies report **higher psychiatric morbidity** in Britain among immigrant Afro-Caribbean and Asian groups than UK-born Europeans, although noted that two studies have found Asians to have lower rates than Europeans. Psychiatric **admission rates** in this study were:

- Increased for the Afro-Caribbean group.
- Similar among the Asian group and UK-born Europeans, except:
- Decreased for the young Asian group (age 16–29 years).

Evidence from studies can be conflicting; the following is a summary of the findings of a selction of these.

Epidemiology of psychosis

Increased rates of schizophrenia are found in:

- Africans.[26]
- Afro-Caribbeans.[27, 28]
- Irish.[29]
- All ethnic groups.[30]
- In addition, **all ethnic groups are more likely to develop psychosis**, but not necessarily schizophrenia[30]

Other evidence:

1. Harrison *et al.*[28] carried out a prospective study in Nottingham of first onset schizophrenia in Afro-Caribbean patients (1984–86) compared to the general population in a World Health Organization study (1978–80). They used the Present State Examination (PSE) and generated DSMIII and ICD9 diagnostic criteria. The denominator used to determine incidence rates was estimated using the 1981 census data (based on the country of birth of the head of household). Incidence rates of schizophrenia were:

   - Increased 12-fold in Afro-Caribbean age groups 16–29 and 30–44.

   - Increased 18-fold in the second-generation Afro-Caribbean age group 16–29.

2. King *et al.*[30] found most **white patients** with schizophrenia were **also** first or second generation **migrants**.

3. Sugarman and Craufurd[31] suggest that the increased frequency of schizophrenia in

Afro-Caribbeans is due to **environmental factors** which are most common in the Afro-Caribbean community, although it is no less familial in them than the rest of the population.

4. McKenzie *et al.*[32] found Afro-Caribbeans to have a better prognosis of psychosis regarding severity of symptoms, course of illness and self-harm.

5. The International Pilot Study of Schizophrenia (IPSS)[4] which covered nine countries, found that the prevalence of schizophrenia was similar in all countries using the Present State Examination (PSE).

6. Sartorius *et al.*[33] conducted a World Health Organization international study in 10 countries of patients making a first contact with any type of helping agency for psychotic symptoms. Patients with schizophrenia had very similar symptoms profiles in all 10 countries. At 2-year follow-up there was a more favourable outcome in developing countries. This may be because of the greater acceptance of symptoms by relatives and friends (thereby reducing high expressed emotion).

In summary, the current focus on schizophrenia in Afro-Caribbeans is misleading as all ethnic minority groups are vulnerable. The most important determinant of mental health of ethnic minorities in Western countries may be the conditions under which they live.[30]

Epidemiology of affective disorders

There are no significant differences in rates of affective disorders for West Indian and Asian groups compared to whites. These disorders are characterised by prominent somatic symptoms in Indians and Pakistanis, as is seen in other developing countries.[18]

Epidemiology of deliberate self-harm and suicide

Suicide rates are:[34]

- High for young Indian females.

- Low for Indian males and elderly Indian females.

- Low for Caribbean immigrants.

Deliberate self-poisoning in West Indians compared to whites shows:[35]

- Age <25 years: rates similar.

- Age > 25 years: rates lower for West Indians.

- West Indians are **more likely** to be young, female and single.

- They are **less likely**:
    - (i) To have previously self-poisoned.
    - (ii) To have a past psychiatric history.
    - (iii) To suffer personality disorder or alcoholism.

Deliberate self-poisoning in Asians compared to whites shows:[36]

- Higher rates for Asian females, but lower for Asian males.

- Asian patients more likely to be young, female and married. Culture conflicts are common.

It has been suggested that deliberate self-harm is a Western culture bound syndrome, but is being adopted by UK-born ethnic groups.[37]

Management in Transcultural Psychiatry

Interpreting services

- These should be used whenever **possible** when the client is not fluent in the same language as the therapist.

- Second language skills can be compromised when ill, lacking in confidence or anxious.

- Miscommunication can occur due to differences in non-verbal communication.

- **Inappropriate to use relatives**, especially children, as interpreters.

- Interpreter needs to speak the same language as the client! (Different dialects exist.)

- Ideal interpreter **respects confidentiality, translates fully and exactly**, and has some health care knowledge.[6]

- How to use an interpreter is detailed in Phelan and Parkman.[38]

Assessment

There is a need for an awareness of the dangers of interpreting symptoms and behaviours across cultural and language differences. Rack[21] describes the diagnostic pitfalls:

- Recognise ethnocentricity, and do not impose own cultural practices on others.

- Consider a person's cultural identity; family structure and organisation, belief systems; personal and social history.

- Avoid stereotyping.

Medication differences

There are racial and ethnic differences in response to psychotropic medication. Possible reasons include:

- Dietary differences.

- Genetic differences in metabolism.

- Environmental factors (e.g. smoking, alcohol intake, exposure to drugs and toxins).

- Cultural factors.

Both genetic and environmental factors could affect the degree of protein binding of drugs. Sensitivity to drug side effects may also vary in different ethnic groups. Lin *et al.*[39] reviewed the literature: **Asians needed lower doses of neuroleptics**, even after body weight was taken into account. Asians and blacks achieved **higher levels** of tricyclic antidepressants than whites. Asians responded to lower doses of lithium, and diazepam was metabolised slower in Asians.

Service provision

Ethnic data

- The **1991 Census** was the first census to record **ethnic origin**. Previous censuses collected information on country of birth. This became an increasingly inaccurate estimate of ethnic minority populations, as the proportion that are British-born increased.

- Ethnic groups constitute 5.9% of the total population of England and Wales. This consists of 1.0% Black Caribbean, 0.4% Black African, 0.4% Black other, 1.7% Indian, 0.9% Pakistani, 0.3% Bangladeshi, 0.3% Chinese, 0.4% Asian other, and 0.6% others.

- Significant differences exist between ethnic groups in numbers, areas of residence, and degree of "clustering". The areas with the highest proportions of ethnic groups are predominantly in London; including 45% and 42% for Brent and Newham boroughs respectively.[40]

- **Ethnic monitoring** has been routine for all hospital admissions in the National Health Service since April 1995, and included in the **Contract Minimum Data Set** from 1994.

- The **ethnic elderly** are a growing and important group. It is a popular myth that they are always looked after by their families. Norman[41] talks of the "Triple Jeopardy" that they may suffer discrimination of old age and ethnicity, as well as lack of access to services.

Relevant history of health care services

- **The National Health Service** was set up in 1948 to serve a fairly homogenous British population. The composition of the population has changed significantly since then, and so have the health needs. The service was designed to be available for all, free at the point of delivery and equal for all. But if a service is not appropriate for a sector of the population, then it is not serving that sector of the population. A health service which maintains a "colour-blind" or "culture-blind" approach is likely to be less sensitive to the health care needs of ethnic minority patients.[6]

- **The Black Report** (report of the Working Group on Inequalities in Health, chaired by Sir Douglas Black in 1977) showed that barriers to access are greater for those in the lower socio-economic

classes. The poorer health experience of the lower
occupational groups applied at all stages of life.
The manual classes make less use of the health
care system, yet need it more.[42]

- **The Inverse Care Law**: the availability of good
  medical care tends to vary inversely with the need
  of the population served.[43]

Equality of service does not mean treating everyone the same,
irrespective of differing needs.

- All people should:
  - (i)   Have **equal access** to the health service via
          appropriate information.
  - (ii) Have services which are both relevant and
          sensitive to their needs.
  - (iii) Be able to use the health service **with ease**,
          and have confidence that they will be treated
          with respect.[44]

- Services need to consider alternative approaches
  to service provision, ensuring that services are
  more **accessible, appropriate, sensitive, flexible
  and accountable**.

- **Training** is vital so that key-workers can recognise
  limitations in their approach and accept alternative
  approaches and models.

- **Consultation with communities** they serve is
  important to build understanding and trust.

- The important contribution of **voluntary
  organisations** operating for ethnic minority
  communities should be recognised, and also that
  their services cannot be effectively replicated

within mainstream settings. Funding policies must secure their structures and ensure their stability and growth.

Role of non-statutory/voluntary agencies and black advocacy groups[45]

- Crucial role in provision of mental health services to multi-ethnic society.

- Offer innovative approaches and meaningful services at grass root level.

- Self-advocacy and collective advocacy about individuals' difficulties with services.

- Looking at alternative ways of understanding emotional distress.

Problems:

- Limited resources and very insecure conditions: resulting in high staff turnover.

- Staff lack training in complex issues surrounding mental health.[46]

Barriers to effective health service provision

- **Lack of information**. Access to services depends upon an adequate knowledge of the service, its purpose, how and when to gain access, and what can be expected from it. To fail to provide such information is to deny access to the service.

- **Communication barriers** (talking in terms that cannot be understood, failing to have trained interpreters on hand, etc.).

- **Lack of understanding**, goodwill and patience among health care staff.

- **Aspects of the service unacceptable to patients**, e.g. mixed wards, washing facilities, religious considerations, food, visiting.

- **Lack of confidence** in the ability of services to understand and meet their needs.

- **Perception of services as alien**, often racist, and not user-friendly.

- Fear that **confidentiality** will not be preserved.

- **Negative past experience** of services.

- Incorrect pronunciation and use of names reduces rapport. Lack of understanding of Asian **naming systems** can lead to multiples sets of notes and its dangers.

Pathways to care: a case of discrimination?

A filtering process operates between the community and the wards of psychiatric hospitals, which is selectively permeable to those with more severe disorders. There is a framework of **five levels and four filters**, where the proportion of potential patients is reduced at each level.[47]

Pathways into psychiatric care can differ according to ethnic origin, e.g. it has been found that **Afro-Caribbeans**:

- Are more likely to be referred by relatives or self.[48]

- Are less likely to be referred by a general practitioner.[49]

- Encounter increased delay in seeking help.[50]

- Receive increased referral by police.[25, 48–51]

In contrast, Cole *et al.*[52] found that ethnicity was **not** a significant determinant of pathway for first onset psychosis, but that police involvement and use of the Mental Health Act were strongly associated with an absence of general practitioner involvement and absence of help-seeking by friends or family.

Studies into the **use of the Mental Health Act** have shown:

- Increased use in Afro-Caribbean patients[25, 49, 53] – 50% of Afro-Caribbeans compared to 10% of non-Afro-Caribbeans.

- Increased use in Asian patients.[25]

- Rates for Asians similar to whites.[53]

- No ethnic difference.[52]

- Black patients are over-represented in **secure units and special hospitals**.[53]

- **Section 136** may be disproportionately used for black patients.[54, 55] Other studies such as Cole *et al.*[52] found no ethnic difference.

Once in contact with the health services, there is evidence that **stereotypes can affect diagnosis and clinical management**:

- Using case vignettes, Lewis *et al.*[56] found Afro-Caribbean patients to be **judged** as potentially more violent, criminal proceedings more appropriate, and more likely to be labelled "cannabis psychosis".

- **Staff may perceive black patients as more dangerous**. Evidence about actual levels of violence are conflicting, but Lawson *et al.*[57] found black in-patients were significantly **less violent** than whites.

- Asians more likely to receive antidepressants.[51]

- There is an increased use of depot neuroleptic medication in Afro-Caribbeans[58, 59] and in older Asian women.[58]

- Depot therapy was initiated after a first episode of

illness significantly more often in Afro-Caribbean patients than in non-Caribbeans.[60] In this study, although there was no overall difference in dosage of neuroleptics, a small subgroup of Afro-Caribbean patients received very much higher peak doses of medication. In three Afro-Caribbean patients, the depot was started on the day of initial contact.

Black patients are **more likely**:

- To receive various physical treatments (major tranquillisers, electroconvulsive therapy) than British-born or white immigrants).[61]
- To receive more "as required" (PRN) medication, and more seclusion and restraint.[62]

They are **less likely**:

- To be referred for psychotherapy.
- To have a broad range of treatments.
- To have recreational and occupational therapy.[62]

Black **and** white immigrants are more likely:

- To receive intramuscular medications.
- To have an out-patient attendance pattern of self-referrals, missed appointments, and to be seen on booked appointments by the most junior members of the therapeutic team.[61]

Black and ethnic minority staff

- They are concentrated in lower grades and less popular specialities – due to discriminatory recruitment and promotion practices.

- They provide a generic service to the white community.

- They are also expected to provide additional services, e.g. interpretation and "expert advice" on minority culture, without further training or promotion.

- Lack of ethnic minority staff adds to the feeling of alienation on hospital wards.[63]

- Racial discrimination against ethnic minority doctors may occur.[64]

- The National Health Service Management Executive (NHSME) has set up a programme of action with the goal *"to achieve equitable representation of minority ethnic groups at all levels in the NHS (including professional staff groups), reflecting the ethnic composition of the local population".*[65]

- Royal College of Psychiatrists[1] has made recommendations about training and recruitment of staff.

Training

Training has a central role in the promotion of race equality in services. The **Royal College of Psychiatrists**, in 1990, stated that *"Transcultural psychiatry is an important element in the education of psychiatrists and the College should give a lead and practical curriculum guidance to tutors".*[1]

Government reforms

Black and ethnic minority health was included in 1988 in the Department of Health's management review of health service performance. The key themes in the development of these health policies are:

- Elimination of racial discrimination.

- Availability of data on black and ethnic minority groups.

- Delivery of appropriate quality services.

- Training of health professionals.

- Information for black and ethnic minority groups on health and health services.

- Recognition of differing patterns of health and disease.[44]

- The **Patient's Charter** emphasises the need for respect of privacy, dignity and religious and cultural beliefs, making this a **statutory requirement**.[66]

- The document *The Health of the Nation* sought to elaborate a strategy for health promotion within the context of the WHO programme "Health for All by the Year 2000".[67]

- Addressing health care inequalities and paying attention to the delivery of psychiatric care in a culturally sensitive manner must be an essential component of this.

Key points

- Have some familiarity with the key features of major ethnic minority groups.

- Be aware of your own culture and the effect this has on your clinical practice.

- Do not stereotype or overgeneralise.

- Be open-minded and willing to learn from patients and communities.

References

[1] Royal College of Psychiatrists. (1990). *Report of the Special Committee on Psychiatric Practice and Training in British Multi-Ethnic Society.* London: Royal College of Psychiatrists.

[2] Fernando S (1991). *Mental Health, Race and Culture.* Macmillan: Hampshire.

[3] Black J (1985). Child health in ethnic minorities. The difficulties of living in Britain. *British Medical Journal,* **290**, 615–617.

[4] *The International Pilot Study of Schizophrenia,* vol. 1. (1973). Geneva: World Health Organization.

[5] Kleinman A (1977). Depression, somatisation and the new 'cross-cultural psychiatry'. *Social Science and Medicine,* **11**, 3–10.

[6] Mares P, Henley A, Baxter C (1985). *Health Care in Multiracial Britain.* Cambridge: Health Education Council and the National Extension College.

[7] Fernando S (ed.) (1995). *Mental Health in a Multi-ethnic Society. A Multidisciplinary Handbook.* London: Routledge.

[8] Lau A (1990). Psychological problems in adolescents from ethnic minorities. *British Journal of Hospital Medicine,* **44**, 201–205.

[9] Leff J (1988). *Psychiatry Around the Globe: a transcultural view.* Gaskell Press: London.

[10] Lipowski Z J (1988). Somatization: the concept and its clinical application. *American Journal of Psychiatry,* **145**, 1358–1368.

[11] Kleinman A, Kleinman J (1985). Somatisation: the interconnections in Chinese society among culture, depressive experiences, and meaning of pain. In *Culture and Depression. Studies in the Anthropology and Cross Culture Psychiatry of Affect and Disorder,* (eds) Kleinman A, Good B. London and Berkeley: University of California Press, pp. 429–490.

[12] Kleinman A (1987). Anthropology and psychiatry. The role of culture in cross-cultural research on illness. *British Journal of Psychiatry,* **151**, 447–454.

[13] Mumford D (1992). Detection of psychiatric disorders among Asian patients presenting with somatic symptoms. *British Journal of Hospital Medicine,* **47**, 202–204.

[14] Littlewood R (1990). From categories to contexts: a decade of the "new cross-cultural psychiatry". *British Journal of Psychiatry,* **156**, 308–327.

[15] Mumford D B, Bevington J T, Bhatnagar K S, Hussain Y, Mirza S, Naraghi M M (1991). The Bradford Somatic Inventory. A multi-ethnic inventory of somatic symptoms reported by anxious and depressed patients in Britain and the Indo-Pakistan subcontinent. *British Journal of Psychiatry,* **158**, 379–386.

[16] Yap P M (1951). Mental disease peculiar to certain cultures: a survey of comparative psychiatry. *Journal of Mental Science,* **97**, 313–327.

[17] Cox J L, Jorsh M S (1992). Transcultural psychiatry. In *The Scientific Basis of Psychiatry,* 2nd edition, (eds) Weller M, Eysenck M. London: W B Saunders.

[18] London M. (1986). Mental illness among immigrant minorities in the United Kingdom (review). *British Journal of Psychiatry,* **149**, 265–273.

[19] Rack P H (1988). Psychiatric and social problems among immigrants. *Acta Psychiatrica Scandinavica,* **78** (suppl 344), 167–173.

[20] Hertz D G (1988). Identity – lost and found: patterns of migration and psychological and psychosocial adjustment of migrants. *Acta Psychiatrica Scandinavica* **78** (suppl 344), 159–165.

[21] Rack P H (1982). *Race, Culture and Mental Disorder* London: Tavistock Publications.

[22] Toffler A. (1970). *Future Shock*. London: Corgi.

[23] Rack P H (1986). Migration and mental illness. In *Transcultural Psychiatry*, (ed.) Cox J L London: Croom Helm.

[24] Littlewood R, Lipsedge M (1988). Psychiatric illness among British Afro-Caribbeans. *British Medical Journal*, **296**, 950–951.

[25] Thomas C S, Stone K, Osborn M, Thomas P F, Fisher M. (1993). Psychiatric morbidity and compulsory admission among UK-born Europeans, Afro-Caribbeans and Asians in central Manchester. *British Journal of Psychiatry*, **163**, 91–99.

[26] Rwegellera G G C (1977). Psychiatric morbidity among West Africans and West Indians living in London. *Psychological Medicine*, **7**, 317–329.

[27] Littlewood R, Lipsedge M (1981) Some social and phenomenological characteristics of psychotic immigrants. *Psychological Medicine*, **11**, 289–302.

[28] Harrison G, Owens D, Holton A, Neilson D, Boot D (1988). A prospective study of severe mental disorder in Afro-Caribbean patients. *Psychological Medicine* 18: 643–657.

[29] Dean G, Downing H, Shelley E (1981). First admissions to psychiatric hospitals in south-east England in 1976 among immigrants from Ireland. *British Medical Journal*, **282**, 1831–1833.

[30] King M, Coker E, Leavey G, Hoare A, Johnson-Sabine E (1994). Incidence of psychotic illness in London: comparison of ethnic groups. *British Medical Journal*, **309**, 1115–1119.

[31] Sugarman P A, Craufurd D (1994). Schizophrenia in the Afro-Caribbean community. *British Journal of Psychiatry*, **164**, 474–480.

[32] McKenzie K, Van Os J, Fahy T, Jones P, Harvey I, Toone B, Murray R (1995). Psychosis with good prognosis in Afro-Caribbean people now living in the United Kingdom. *British Medical Journal*, **311**, 1325–1328.

[33] Sartorius N, Jablensky A, Korten A, Ernberg G, Anker M, Cooper J E, Day R (1986). Early manifestations and first-contact incidence of schizophrenia in different cultures. *Psychological Medicine*, **16**, 909–928.

[34] Raleigh V S, Balarajan R (1992). Suicide and self burning among Indians and West Indians in England and Wales. *British Journal of Psychiatry*, **161**, 365–368.

[35] Merrill J, Owens J (1987). Ethnic differences in self-poisoning. A comparison of West Indian and white groups. *British Journal of Psychiatry*, **150**, 765–768.

[36] Merrill J, Owens J (1986). Ethnic differences in self-poisoning: a comparison of Asian and white groups. *British Journal of Psychiatry*, **148**, 708–712.

[37] Merrill J, Owens J (1988). Self-poisoning among four immigrant groups. *Acta Psychiatrica Scandinavica*, **77**, 77–80.

[38] Phelan M, Parkman S (1995). How to do it. Work with an interpreter. *British Medical Journal*, **311**, 555–557.

[39] Lin K M, Poland R E, Lesser I R (1986). Ethnicity and psychopharmacology. *Culture Medicine and Psychiatry*, **10**, 151–165.

40   Balarajan R, Raleigh V S (1992). The ethnic populations of England and Wales: the 1991 census. *Health Trends,* **24**, 113–116.

41   Norman A (1985). *Triple Jeopardy. Growing Old in a Second Homeland.* London: Centre for Policy on Ageing.

42   Townsend P, Davidson N (1982). Inequality in the availability and use of the health service. In *Inequalities in Health: The Black Report,* (eds) Townsend P, Davidson, N. Penguin.

43   Hart J T (1971). 'The inverse care law'. *Lancet,* 27 February, 405–412.

44   Hopkins A, Bahl V (eds) (1993). *Access to Health Care for People from Black and Ethnic Minorities.* London: Royal College of Physicians.

45   Sassoon M, Lindow V (1995). Consulting and empowering Black mental health system users. In *Mental Health in a Multi-Ethnic Society. A Multidisciplinary Handbook,* (ed.) Fernando S. London: Routledge.

46 Ahmed T, Webb-Johnson A (1995). Voluntary groups. In *Mental Health in a Multi-Ethnic Society. A Multi-Disciplinary Handbook,* (ed.) Fernando S. London: Routledge.

47   Goldberg D, Huxley P (1992). *Common Mental Disorders. A Bio-Social Model.* Routledge: London.

48   Rwegellera G G C (1980). Differential use of psychiatric services by West Indians, West Africans and English in London. *British Journal of Psychiatry,* **137**, 428–432.

49   Owens D, Harrison G, Boot D (1991). Ethnic factors in voluntary and compulsory admissions. *Psychological Medicine,* **21**, 185–196.

50   Harrison G, Holton A, Neilson D, Owens D, Boot D, Cooper J (1989). Severe mental disorder in Afro-Caribbean patients: some social, demographic and service factors. *Psychological Medicine,* **19**, 683–696.

51   Perera R, Owens D G, Johnstone E C (1991). Disabilities and circumstances of schizophrenia patients – a follow-up study. Ethnic aspects. A comparison of three matched groups. *British Journal of Psychiatry,* **159**, (suppl 13), 40–42.

52   Cole E, Leavey G, King M, Johnson-Sabine E, Hoar A (1995). Pathways to care for patients with a first episode of psychosis. A comparison of ethnic groups. *British Journal of Psychiatry,* **167**, 770–776.

53   McGovern D, Cope R (1987). The compulsory detention of males of different ethnic groups, with special reference to offender patients. *British Journal of Psychiatry,* **150**, 505–512.

54   Dunn J, Fahy T A (1990). Police admissions to a psychiatric hospital: demographic and clinical differences between ethnic groups. *British Journal of Psychiatry,* **156**, 373–378.

55   Pipe R, Bhat A, Matthews B, Hampstead J (1991). Section 136 and African/Afro-Caribbean minorities. *International Journal of Social Psychiatry,* **37**, 14–23.

56   Lewis G, Croft-Jeffreys C, David A (1990). Are British psychiatrists racist? *British Journal of Psychiatry,* **157**, 410–415.

57   Lawson W B, Yesavage J A, Werner P D (1984). Race, violence and psychopathology. *Journal of Clinical Psychiatry,* **45**, 294–297.

58   Glover G, Malcolm G (1988). The prevalence of depot neuroleptic treatment among West Indians and Asians in the London borough of Newham. *Social Psychiatry and Psychiatric Epidemiology,* **23**, 281–284.

59 Lloyd K, Moodley P (1991). Psychotropic medication and ethnicity: an inpatient survey. *Social Psychiatry and Psychiatric Epidemiology*, **27**, 95–101.

60 Chen E Y H, Harrison G, Standen P J (1991). Management of first episode psychotic illness in Afro-Caribbean patients. *British Journal of Psychiatry*, **158**, 517–522.

61 Littlewood R, Cross S (1980). Ethnic minorities and psychiatric services. *Sociology of Health and Illness*, **2**, 194–201.

62 Flagerty J A, Meagher R (1980). Measuring racial bias in inpatient treatment. *American Journal of Psychiatry*, **137**, 679–682.

63 Fernando S (1988). *Race and Culture in Psychiatry*. London: Croom Helm.

64 Esmail A, Everington S (1993). Racial discrimination against doctors from ethnic minorities. *British Medical Journal*, **306**, 691–692.

65 NHS Management Executive, Department of Health (1993). *Ethnic Minority Staff in the NHS: A Programme for Action*. London: HMSO.

66 Department of Health. (1991). *The Patient's Charter*. London: HMSO.

67 Department of Health. (1992). *The Health of the Nation – a Strategy for Health in England*. London: HMSO.

Chapter 12

Setting up and auditing an old age psychiatry service

Stephen Curran

Introduction

The document **Mental Health of the Nation; the Contribution of Psychiatry**[1] is the executive response by the Royal College of Psychiatrists to the Secretary of State's strategy for health in England. This document highlights that only through well organised services can good quality care be delivered to those most in need. In addition, if a service is well planned it can provide better quality care for a greater number at no additional cost. The document also specifically identifies elderly psychiatric patients as a "*vulnerable group*". The principal aim of an old age psychiatry service must be to meet the needs "*of the old people in its community*". It should be concerned with the development of a comprehensive range of services for the assessment, treatment and care of elderly mentally ill patients in the community and not just those in hospital.[2]

There are many different service styles, e.g. joint assessment wards (with Medicine for the Elderly), those only dealing with demented patients, and services with a heavy teaching responsibility, such as academic units. In the "ideal" service, all patients referred with psychiatric morbidity within a defined population should be seen with the aim of maintaining people at home for as long as possible.[3]

Psychiatric services for the elderly cannot be planned rationally at a **local level** unless several types of information are considered in the planning process. These include:

- The number of people at risk.

- The incidence and prevalence of various psychiatric problems in different age groups.

- Other demographic factors such as social class, quality of housing, provision of other services, etc.

- Degree of social isolation.

- Poverty.

- Ethnicity.

- Gender distribution.

- Existing local provision.

In addition, major mood, paranoid and neurotic disorders are at least as common in old age as in younger adults. The prevalence of dementia gradually increases with increasing age with 20% of those over 80 years of age showing evidence of dementia.[1] Other important problems in this age group include physical ill health and numerous losses, e.g. bereavement and loss of income. It is important to have services giving care of the highest quality, from well-trained practitioners providing a comprehensive service. It is also particularly important to involve the families of patients and to foster a close working relationship with other health care professionals. Central to the provision of this care is the multidisciplinary team (MDT).

Organising an Old Age Psychiatry Service

Services for elderly mentally ill patients have traditionally been provided by units serving a population of a defined catchment area. However, there are wide variations in terms of size, structure, organisation and level of resources, and this is due to a number of factors as described above. The following general principles need to be taken into account when setting up an old age psychiatry service:

- There must be adequate provision of **bridging finance** to ensure satisfactory community services are in place before established services are withdrawn.

- Good levels of communication between **purchasers and providers** must be established.

The fundamental unit of service delivery is the **multidisciplinary team** (MDT). A consultant works with, and leads, a team including:

- Ward nurses.

- Community Psychiatric Nurses (CPNs).

- Clinical psychologists.

- Social workers.

- Occupational therapists.

- Other health care professionals.

Staffing

For each clinical team, the Royal College recommends that there should be between two and six Community Psychiatric Nurses. Acute wards require a minimum of one nurse per 1.2 beds and on long stay wards one nurse per 1.5 beds.[4]

Guidelines for other health care professionals (e.g. social workers) are less clearly defined. Provision of consultant manpower should recognise the demands of providing a modern, community-based psychiatric service of high quality with 1.6 consultants per 100 000 of the general population. More specifically, the current requirement for consultant manpower should increase from the present level to one consultant for every 10 000 patients aged 65 or over.

Bed provision

The service should be managed in an integrated way in the same provider units as either general psychiatry or medicine for the elderly (or both). The following facilities will be needed:

- **10/10 000 acute in-patient beds** for the assessment, investigation and treatment of patients with problems too severe to be managed elsewhere. This may need to be increased depending on local circumstances (e.g. if the service deals with pre-senile patients or takes "graduate" chronic psychotics). All acute beds should be on a general hospital site. A proportion of these should be for functional patients (1/3) and the remainder for dementia assessment.

- **25–30/10 000 long stay beds** (including respite) for elderly patients suffering from long-term, often progressive disorders, particularly dementia. These may be situated on a general hospital site or elsewhere. However, they require a full range of expert professional input including consultant time, rehabilitation, training and education. It is often useful to have the day hospital geographically near to these beds.

- These figures are based on the assumption that 16% of the population are over 64. If this figure increases, for what ever reason, local services will need to increase accordingly. Only a small proportion of long stay beds need be devoted to "functional" patients.[1]

- In addition to these, approximately **6.5/10 000 functional** and **30/10 000 dementia day hospital places** will be needed.[5]

Over the next few years, a rapid increase in the "old old" with all the problems associated with this (medical, psychiatric and social) will put further pressure on old age psychiatry services, with the need for further revisions and recommendations.[6] It is also important that the service is able to liaise effectively with other health care professionals including:

- Primary health care.
- Geriatric medicine.
- Other medical services.
- Local Authority services.
- Voluntary and private sector.

For each part of the services (e.g. acute in-patient ward, long stay ward, day hospital, community services) it may be useful to draw up an **operational policy** after consultation with all the appropriate staff, which clearly defines issues such as aims, mechanism for referral, details of assessment, etc.

Consultant responsibilities

The consultant old age psychiatrist plays a central role in delivering care to elderly people with a mental illness. When setting up an old age psychiatry service the issues discussed above need to be taken into account. Attention will also have to be given to areas such as the **location** of various units (e.g. day hospital, long stay wards, out-patient clinics), **suitability of buildings, availability of facilities** (e.g. biochemistry and haematology) and **availability of rooms** for staff, both for personal use and team meetings. **Time** will also need to be planned to give to junior medical, nursing and secretarial staff. Finally, **adequate** and **flexible transport facilities** need to be available to bring patients efficiently to out-patients, day hospital, etc.

In addition:

- The service should have a reasonable number of patients to care for (not too many and not too few).

- Time needs to be devoted to personal development, continuing medical education and personal research.

- Once an old age psychiatry service has been set up it will be necessary to ensure that the service as a whole, and individual parts of it, are working well. This is achieved through a variety of mechanisms including the **audit cycle**.

Medical Audit

The terms "medical audit" and "clinical audit" are often used interchangeably. However, clinical audit might be considered to cover all aspects of clinical care whereas medical audit relates to practices initiated directly by doctors.[7]

Medical audit can be defined as "*the systematic, critical analysis of the quality of medical care, including the procedures used for diagnosis and treatment, the use of resources, and the resulting outcomes and quality of life for the patient*".[8] There have been some useful reviews of audit,[9–12] and some of the important issues are now briefly discussed.

Seven principles of medical audit have been defined by Shaw and Costain:[7]

1. Health Authorities and medical staff should **explicitly define** their respective responsibilities for the **quality** of patient care.

2. Medical staff should **organise themselves** in order to fulfil responsibilities for audit and for taking action to improve clinical practice.

3. Each hospital and speciality should agree a **regular programme** of audit in which doctors in all grades participate.

4. The process of audit should be **relevant, objective, quantified, repeatable** and able to **effect appropriate change** in the organisation of the service and clinical practice.

5. Clinicians should be provided with the **resources** for medical audit.

6. The process and outcome of medical audit should be **documented** and **distributed** to those to whom it is relevant.

7. Medical audit should be subject to **evaluation**.

Medical audit differs from more traditional reviews, such as ward rounds, in the following ways:

- Explicit criteria for good practice are stated.

- It quantifies current patterns of practice.

- It compares individual performances with peers.

- It leads to agreed action for improvement.

- It requires specific documentation.[12]

In addition, medical audit involves a **cycle** of activities (Fig. 12.1), and failure to complete the cycle is the commonest cause of "failed" audit.

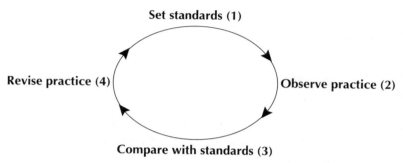

Fig. 12.1 The audit cycle.

The original standards may be set from a variety of sources. Once set, these can be compared with observed practice and in the light of this comparison, practice can be revised. The original standards may be based on observation of one's own practice, national guidelines, Royal College guidelines, literature reviews, consensus statements or "current" practice. A specific intervention should be assessed by using a **defined outcome** (e.g. reduced waiting time) and a good outcome measure should be **valid, specific and precisely defined**. It should also be possible to measure it **objectively** and it should be **appropriate** to one's practice.

Getting started in audit

- Find topics that are of interest to the group and are clinically relevant.
- Start with something simple.
- Be selective.
- Avoid massive data collection – they will take too long to analyse, and may not address the specific questions you want to answer.
- Make sure your group is committed.

Choosing what to audit

The following framework may help identify a particular aspect of the old age psychiatry service to audit:

- **Access to services**:
    (i)   Waiting lists.
    (ii) Travel times.
    (iii) Cross boundary flow.
    (iv) Home visits.

- **Relevance of services**: achievement of targets. Does the team provide the range of services that is required?

- **Effectiveness of services**: are interventions effective? What is the outcome clinically in depression, paraphrenia, etc.?

- **Equity of services**: fairness and equitable access to services.

- **Acceptability of services**:
    (i)   Patients.
    (ii) Relatives.
    (iii) Purchasers.

- **Efficiency of services**: unit costs, time spent travelling, in-patient stays, etc.

Sources of material for use in audit

A variety of sources for data exist which can be used in audit including:

- Questionnaires (patients, relatives, staff). What is their opinion about the service?

- Routinely collected data (e.g. are electroconvulsive therapy consent forms adequately documented?).

- Patients' records (adequately filled in admission documentation, etc.).
- Letters/request forms.
- Clinical specimens. (Are these requested? If so, are the results clearly recorded in the notes?).
- Video recordings (consultation styles).
- Computer-based information.
- Libraries.

Audit method

There are also a number of different audit methods including:

- Criteria-based audit.
- Adverse occurrence screening.
- Critical incident review.
- Patient survey.
- Peer review.

In terms of auditing an old age psychiatry service, **criteria-based audit** is probably the most useful. This method identifies measurable criteria and defines specific standards for an aspect of care which can then be compared with what actually happens in practice. It has a number of advantages and disadvantages.[13]

Advantages of criteria-based audit

- Quality is explicitly expressed and agreed before audit.
- It makes actual practice explicit.
- Data collection can be fast.
- Agreed standards can be achieved.

- Improvement can be measured.

- Screeners can be non-medical.

Disadvantages of criteria based audit

- Accurate clinical indices are needed.

- Agreeing standards can be difficult.

- May require review of a large amount of data, e.g. case notes.

- Time consuming and difficult if done by only one person.

The audit meeting

The audit should be organised through the **audit meeting** and a number of elements contribute to its success. These include:

- **Organisation**: one person should be designated for organising meetings (Lead Clinician).

- **Timing**: half day per month is usual.

- **Attendance**: minimum of 70% of all grades.

- **Supporting documentation**: minutes, case notes, etc.

- **Group size**: variable but usually 3–15.

Using these general principles, it is possible to set up an audit group, and audit a part of the old age psychiatry service which the clinical team feel would benefit from careful examination and discussion.

Key points

- Setting up an old age psychiatry service requires careful planning and should be developed at the local level. The service should include a range of in-patient and out-patient assessments and treatments.

- The Royal College guidelines provide clear suggestions for the structure and manning of such a service.

- A multidisciplinary team approach forms an effective basis for service provision. Staff training, including continuing professional development, is an important feature of an effective team.

- The audit cycle provides a key element for the review and improvement of clinical services.

- Audit should be specific, objective and be reviewed within the audit meeting. Criteria-based audit makes actual practice explicit. Agreed standards can be prepared and improvement can be measured.

References

[1] *Mental Health of the Nation; The Contribution of Psychiatry; A Report of the President's Working Group.* (1992). Council report CR16. London: Royal College of Psychiatrists.

[2] Pitt B (1992). *Psychogeriatrics; An Introduction to the Psychiatry of Old Age.* London: Churchill Livingstone.

[3] Arie T, Isaacs A D (1978). The development of psychiatric services for the elderly in Britain. In *Studies in Geriatric Psychiatry*, (eds) Isaacs A D, Post F. Chichester: John Wiley and Sons, pp. 241–261.

[4] *Addendum on Nurse Staffing* (1977). London: Royal College of Psychiatrists

[5] *Interim Guidelines for Regional Advisors on Consultant Posts in Psychiatry of Old Age* (1979). London: Royal College of Psychiatrists.

[6] Brothwood J (1971). The organisation and development of services for the

aged with special reference to the mentally ill. In *Recent Developments in Psychogeriatrics*, (eds) Kay D W K, Walk A. *British Journal of Psychiatry*. Ashford: Headley Brothers Ltd., pp. 99–112.

[7] Shaw C D, Costain D W (1989). Guidelines for medical audit; seven principles. *British Medical Journal*, **299**, 498–499.

[8] Department of Health (1989). *Working for Patients*, Working Paper 6, Command 555. HMSO: London.

[9] Mugford M, Banfield P, O'Hanlon M (1991). Effects of feedback of information on clinical practice; a review. *British Medical Journal*, **303**, 398–402.

[10] Russell I T, Wilson B J (1992). Audit; the third clinical science. *Quality in Health Care*, **1**, 51–55.

[11] Bowden D, Walshe K (1992). When medical audit starts to count. *British Medical Journal*, **303**, 101–103.

[12] *Making Medical Audit Effective* (1992). London: Joint Centre for Education in Medicine.

[13] Shaw C D (1990). Criterion based audit. *British Medical Journal*, **300**, 649–651.

Index

Abuse in childhood
  assessment and treatment, 115–116
  effects of, 117–118
  epidemiology, 116–117
  factors influencing effects, prognosis and
      planning of treatment, 118–120
  interventions, 120–123
  general principles, 120–121
  individual work, 121–122
Activity, chronic fatigue
      syndrome, 109–110
Acute in-patient beds, elderly patients, 232
Admission to hospital
  Afro-Caribbean and Asian groups, 210
  anorexia nervosa, 81–82
  children, 132
  chronic psychiatric difficulties, 189
  somatisation, 100
  see also Discharged patients and also Mental
      hospitals
Adolescents, physically abused, 117
Affect, lexicon of, 204
Affective disorders, 26, 149, 152–153
  epidemiology, ethnic minority groups, 212
Afro-Caribbean patients
  morbidity rates, 210
  pathways to care, 219, 220
  schizophrenia, 211–212
  stereotyping, clinical management, 220–221
Agranulocytosis, 33, 34
Alcohol abuse, schizophrenia, 26–27
Alzheimer's disease, 149, 154–155
  familial, 155–156
Amitriptyline, 19, 170–171
Amyloid cascade hypothesis, 154
Amyloid plaques, 154
Amyloid precursor protein (APP), 154
  mutations, 155
Anger management, 175
Anorexia nervosa (AN)
  admitting to hospital, 81–82

cognitive therapy, 67–75
end stage, 79–81
epidemiology, 66–67
key features, 65–66
people affected, 69–70
specific points in treatment, 77–79
stressors and relationships, 75–76
Antecedent modification, 125
Anti-psychiatry movement, 187
Anticipation, phenomenon of, 157–158
Anxiety
  cognitive models, 51–52, 54–55
  negative automatic thoughts, 44
  non-Western societies, 204
  with personality disorder, outcome studies,
      181
Anxious preoccupation, 51
Apolipoprotein E, Alzheimer's disease, 155–156
Asian patients
  lithium, 215
  morbidity rates, 210
  naming systems, 219
  neuroleptics, 215, 220
Assertiveness training, 175–176
Asylums, historical review, 185–188
At-risk register, 120
Audit cycle, 236
Auditing, old age psychiatry service, 234–240
  audit meeting, 239
  getting started, 236
  methods, 238–239
  seven principles of, 235
  sources of material, 237–238
  what to audit, 237
Autism, 130
Aversive techniques, behaviour therapy, 126
Avoidance behaviours, 52, 54, 55, 56
Axis 1 and Axis 2 disorder co-morbidity, 178

'Back from the future' letter, 73–74
Bacteriophage vectors, 144

Batch living, 186
Beck, Aaron, 42
  negative cognitive triad, 47
Behaviour therapy
  child psychiatry, 124–126
  cognitive *see* Cognitive behaviour therapy
Behavioural
  analysis, personality disorders, 173–174
  regimes, anorexia, 81–82
Benzodiazepines
  personality disorders, 179
  somatisation, 101
  treatment resistant schizophrenia, 34
Beta-blockers, anxiety, 101
Binary management, 186
Bingeing, 69, 72
Black advocacy groups, 218
Black Report, 216–217
Bodily sensations, heightened response, 51, 52,
    53, 54
  see also Somatisation
Body perceptions, altered in anorexia nervosa,
    78
Borderline personality disorder (BPD)
  DSM-IV diagnostic criteria, 169
  haloperidol and phenelzine, 170
  individual psychotherapy, 176, 177
  MAOIs, 171
  tricyclic antidepressants, 170–171
Bradford somatic inventory, 205
Brief solution focused family therapy, 137
Briquet's syndrome, 94, 104
Bulimia nervosa (BN)
  cognitive therapy, 67–75
  emotional and physical impact, 72–73
  epidemiology, 66–67
  key features, 66
  multi-impulsive patients, 82–83
  with personality disorder, 178
    outcome studies, 180–181
  specific points in treatment
    avoiding craving, 84–85
    identifying 'vicious cycle of bulimia',
      83–84
  stressors and relationships, 75–76

Candidate genes, 148, 149, 152, 153
  dopamine receptor genes, 151
Carbamazepine
  personality disorders, 172–173
  treatment resistant
    depression, 18–19
    schizophrenia, 27
Care programme approach (CPA), 193–194
  application, 194
  schizophrenia, 37–38

Caring for People, White Paper, 188–189, 193
Case conferences, child abuse, 120–121
Catastrophic thoughts, 53, 56
  challenging, 54–55
  see also Cognitive distortions *and also*
     Negative automatic thoughts (NATs)
Category fallacy, 202
Census, 1991: 210, 215
Chaining, behaviour therapy, 125
Child abuse team, 120
Child psychiatry
  abuse in childhood, 115–123
  family therapy, 119, 123, 132–138
  practical treatment in, 124–132
    individual psychotherapy, 130–131
Child sexual abuse accommodation syndrome,
    118
Chlorpromazine
  children, 129
  eating disorders, 77
  treatment resistant schizophrenia, 30
Chromosomal
  abnormalities
    familial Alzheimer's disease, 155–156
    Huntington's disease, 158
    manic depression, 153
    mental retardation, 159, 160, 161
    schizophrenia, 150–152
    X chromosome, 153, 157
  divisions, 151
Chronic fatigue syndrome, 102–112
  aetiology, 103–104
  diagnosis/classification, 105–106
  historical background, 102–103
  management, 108–112
  presentation, 107–108
  prognosis, 112
Clomipramine, 180
Cloning
  DNA, 143–144
  positional, 148–149
Clozapine, 33–34
Clozapine Patient Monitoring System (CPMS),
    33–34
Clunis inquiry, 195
Cluster B personality disorders, 177
Cluster C personality disorder, 177, 178
Cognitive behaviour therapy, 41–64
  child psychiatry, 131
  chronic fatigue syndrome, 111
  eating disorders, 67–75, 180
  parent training, child abuse, 122
  somatisation, 99, 101
  theoretical basis, 42–44
  treatment resistant depression, 22
    schizophrenia, 36
  treatment strategies, 44–47

Cognitive behaviour therapy (*cont*)
    gathering information, 45–46
    patient selection, 44
    style of therapy, 44–45
    teaching new skills, 46–47
Cognitive distortions
    depression, 47–50
    eating disorders, 74–75
    table of, 48
    see also Catastrophic thoughts *and also*
        Negative automatic thoughts (NATs)
Collaborative empiricism, 45
Collective responsibility, mental health teams,
    197
Comfort eating, 72
Community care, 185–200
    alternatives to hospitalisation studies,
        191–192
    concept of, 188–192
        criticism, 192–193
    efforts to improve, 193–196
    the future, 197–198
    schizophrenia, 37
Community Mental Health Centre movement,
    US, 188
Community supervision order, 194
    see also Supervision registers
Community, as term, 188
Complementary therapies, 205
Compulsions, 57, 58, 59
Confidentiality, 196
Consultant responsibilities, old age psychiatrist,
    233–234
Contingency management, behaviour therapy,
    125–126
Cosmid vectors, 144
Covert sensitisation, 126
Criteria-based audit, 238–239
Critical discussion, 3
Cultural
    differences, illness behaviour, 91
    focus on food, 70–71
    identity, 214
    see also Transcultural psychiatry
Culture
    definition, 202
    shock, 208
    syndromes bound with, 206, 213
Cytogenic abnormalities, screening, 148

D2 blockade, schizophrenia, 30
Day patient units
    child, 132
    dementia, 233
Dean and Gadd study, intensive home
    treatment, 192
Definitions in essays, 3

Deinstitutionalisation, 187, 188
Dementia
    Alzheimer's disease, 149, 154–155
        familial, 155–156
    day hospital places, 233
    prevalence, 230
Department of Health, review of health service
    performance, 222–223
Depot therapy, 189, 220–221
Depression
    in children, treatment, 130
    cognitive model, 47–50
    negative automatic thoughts, 43
    non-Western societies, 204
    with personality disorder, 177–178
        implications for treatment, 178–179
        outcome studies, 181
    treatment resistant, 13–23
        apparent treatment failure, 14–15
        management, 17–22
        pharmacological treatments, 16–17
        potential consequences, 15–16
        risk factors, 15
        role of psychosocial factors, 22
Desensitisation
    behaviour therapy, 125
    to fear, 56–57
Desmopressin, 129
Dexamphetamine, 129
Diagnosis
    differential, depressive disorders, 14–15
    transcultural psychiatry
        pitfalls, 209
        questionnaires, 205
Diaries, eating, 69
Diazepam, Asian patients, 215
Diet, child psychiatry, 131–132
Differential reinforcement, 124
Discharged patients, 197
    long-stay, 190–191
Disease and illness, 90
DNA
    amplified by PCR, 145–146
    cloning, 143–144
    labelling, 143
    libraries, 144
    microsatellite, 147–148
Dopamine D2 receptor gene, 151
Double depression, 15, 171
Down's syndrome and Alzheimer's disease,
    155
Downward arrow technique, NATs,
    50
Drama therapy, 128
Drug abuse
    dyssocial personality disorder, 178
    schizophrenia, 26–27

DSM-IV, personality disorder
    classification, 167
    diagnostic criteria, 169
Dyad work, marital therapy, 131
Dyssocial personality disorder, 176, 178
Dysthymia, 171, 172
    with personality disorder, outcome studies,
        181

Eating disorders, 65–88
    cognitive therapy, 67–75
    epidemiology, 66–67
    multi-impulsive patients, 82–83
    with personality disorder, 178
    stress and relationships, 75–76
Electroconvulsive therapy (ECT)
    treatment resistant
    depression, 20
    schizophrenia, 35
Electrophoresis, 146
    agarose gel, 142, 143
Ellis, Albert, 42
Emotion
    high expressed, 27–28, 36–37, 76, 212
    language of, 204
Enuresis, 125, 128–129
Environmental factors, child abuse, 119
Epidemic neuromyasthenia *see* Chronic fatigue
        syndrome
Epidemiology
    child abuse, 116–117
    eating disorders, 66–67
    ethnic minority groups
        affective disorders, 212
        psychosis, 211–212
        self-harm and suicide, 213
    personality disorders, 168
    transcultural psychiatry, 209–213
Essay technique
    blindspots, 10
    essay spotting, 2
    preparation, 1–2
    role of examiner, 9
    structure, 3–5, 9
    what not to do, 10
    what to do, 9–10
    worked examples, 5–9
Ethnic data, 215–216
Ethnic minorities, 202, 206
    population size, 210
    staff, 221–222
Ethnic monitoring, 216
Ethnicity, 202
Ethnocentricism, 203, 214
Exposure
    behaviour therapy, 125
    fears, 56–57

obsessional thoughts, 59
Extinction, behaviour therapy, 125

Familial Alzheimer's disease, 155–156
Families
    factors in child abuse, 119
    high expressed emotion, 27–28, 212
        interventions, 36–37
Family therapy, 132–138
    child abuse, 119, 123
    eating disorders, 75–76
    effectiveness of, 137–138
    formal, 133
    schools of, 134–137
    uses of, 133–134
Family tree construction, 137
Fears, exposure to, 56–57
Finkelhor's model of dynamics, 117–118
Fluorescent *in-situ* hybridisation (FISH),
        144–145
Fluoxetine
    children, 129
    high dose, bulimia nervosa, 86
    personality disorders, 171–172
Focused psychological treatments, personality
        disorders, 173–176
Follow-up after discharge, 189
    long-stay patients, 190–191
Food
    craving, avoiding, 84–85
    cultural focus on, 70–71
    as symbol of love, 71–72
Fragile X syndrome (FRAX-A), 157–158

γ amino butyric acid (GABA) receptor gene, 152
Genes, isolation of mutated, 142–149
Genetic markers, linkage analysis, 148
Gilles de la Tourette syndrome, 130
Goffman, Irving, 186
Group therapy
    child psychiatry, 127–128
        child abuse, 122
    personality disorders, 176

Haley, Jay, 135–136
Haloperidol
    children, 129, 130
    personality disorder, 170
    treatment resistant schizophrenia, 27, 30
Hawthorn effect, 191
The Health of the Nation, White Paper, 223
    see also Mental Health of the Nation
        document
Health service
    barriers to effective, 218–219
    Department of Health review, 222–223
    equality of, 217

Health Service (*cont*)
  pathways to care, 219–221
  see also National Health Service
Helicoptering, 3–4, 6–7
High dose neuroleptics, 30
  dangers, 31
  Royal College Consensus statement, 31–33
High expressed emotion, 212
  eating disorders, 76
  schizophrenia, 27–28, 36–37
High risk groups, 194, 195
History, patient
  eating, 68
  somatisation, 96–97
HIV seropositivity, 178
Hospitals, mental *see* Mental hospitals
Huntington's disease, 158
Hyperkinetic disorder, treatment, 129
Hyperventilation, 52, 56
Hypochondriasis, 94
  cognitive model, 60
Hypothyroidism, sub-clinical, 19
Hysteria, 94

ICD-10, classification of personality disorder,
  167
Icelandic disease *see* Chronic fatigue syndrome
Ideas, overvalued, 67
Illness behaviour, 91–92
  abnormal, 93
  somatisation, 95–96
  transcultural approaches, 204–206
Imipramine, 128, 129
Impulsivity, 172, 174–175
In-patient units, children, 132
Inborn errors of metabolism, 161
Individual psychotherapy
  child psychiatry, 130–131
    abuse in childhood, 121–122
  personality disorders, 176–177
Inherited psychiatric disease, 149–161
Inmate role, 186
  see also Sick role
Institutional perspective, 186
Intensive home treatment study, 192
International Pilot Study of Schizophrenia,
  212
Interpreters, use of, 214
Interviewing, motivational, 73–74
Inverse Care Law, 217
IQ scores, mental retardation, 159

Kelly, George, 41

L-tryptophan, 16, 19
Labelling DNA, 143
Laxatives, eating disorders, 68, 74

Legal system, consequences of in child abuse,
  123
Liaison psychiatry, 89–114
Light therapy, 21
Linkage analysis, 146–148, 149
Lithium
  Asian patients, 215
  personality disorders, 172
  treatment resistant
    depression, 16, 18
    schizophrenia, 35
Litigation, 196
Lod scores, 147, 152
Long stay beds, elderly patients, 232–233

Marks, Isaac, 55
Mechanic, David, 91
  10 determinants of illness behaviour, 91–92
Medanes, C, 135–136
Media
  chronic fatigue syndrome, 111
  murders by mentally ill, 192
Medical audit *see* Auditing, old age psychiatry
    service
Medication differences, ethnic responses, 215
Mental health, Eastern and Western views, 203
Mental health legislation, 197–198
  Mental Health Act, 187
    tube feeding, 79–80
    use of in pathways to care, ethnic minority
      groups, 219–220
  see also NHS and Community Care Act,
    1990
Mental Health of the Nation document, 229
Mental hospitals, 185–186
  bed occupancy in UK and US, 186
  bed provision, elderly patients, 232–233
  closure program, 188
  disenchantment with, 186–187
  see also Admission to hospital
Mental retardation, 158–161
  autosomal dominant and recessive conditions,
    160
  Down's syndrome, 155
  Fragile X syndrome (FRAX-A), 157
Microsatellite DNA, 147–148
Migration, 206, 207
  difficulties caused by, 208
  reasons for, 207–208
  stages of adjustment to, 208–209
Milan School of family therapy, 136–137
Minuchin, Salvador, 134–135
Misdiagnosis, transcultural psychiatry, 209
Moclobamide
  children, 129
  treatment resistant depression, 16
Modelling, behaviour therapy, 125

Molecular genetics, 141
  inherited psychiatric disease, 149–161
  isolation of mutated genes, 142–149
Monoamine oxidase inhibitors (MAOIs)
  personality disorders, 171
  somatisation, 101
  treatment resistant depression, 16, 18
  and tricyclic combination, 19
Motivational interviewing, 73–74
Multidisciplinary team (MDT), old age
    psychiatry service, 230, 231
Murders, mentally ill in community, 192–193
Mutated gene isolation, molecular genetic
    techniques, 142–149
Myalgia–eosinophilia syndrome, 19
Myalgic encephalomyelitis (ME) *see* Chronic
    fatigue syndrome

National Health Service, 187, 216
  Management Executive (NHSME), 222
  NHS and Community Care Act, 1990: 193
  see also Health service
Negative automatic thoughts (NATs), 43–44, 47
  challenging, 46, 49
  see also Catastrophic thoughts
Negative reinforcement, 126
Neglect in childhood, somatisation, 96
Neurasthenia, 103
Neurofibrillary tangles, 154
Neuroleptics, 77, 129
  Asian patients, 215, 220
  depot, Afro-Caribbean patients, 220–221
  personality disorders, 170
  psychotic depression, 20
  schizophrenia
    altering dose, 29–33
    atypical antipsychotic drugs, 33–34
Neuroses with personality disorder, 177,
    178–179
"Newcastle cocktail", 19
NHS and Community Care Act, 1990, 193
Northern blotting, 143

Obsessions, 57, 58, 59
Obsessive–compulsive disorder (OCD), 57–59
  cognitive conceptualisation, 58
  with personality disorder, outcome studies,
    180
Old age psychiatry service, 229–230
  medical audit, 234–240
  organising, 231–234
Organic delusional disorders, 26
Overvalued ideas, 67
Oxford criteria, chronic fatigue syndrome,
    105–106

Pad and bell devices, behaviour therapy, 125

Pain, re-interpreting source of, 60
Palazzoli, Selvini, 136–137
Panic
  cognitive model, 52–53
  with personality disorder, outcome studies,
    181
Paranoid schizophrenic illness, 152
Parents
  factors in child abuse, 119
  parent training, 122–123, 126–127
Patient's Charter, 223
Pemoline, 129
Personality disorders, 165–184
  chronological development of concept,
    165–166
  co-morbidity, 177–179
  current classifications, 167
  epidemiology, 168
  treatment, 168–177
Phenelzine
  personality disorders, 170, 171
  treatment resistant depression, 19
Phenothiazines, 186
Phenotype, inaccuracies in definition, 150
Phenylketonuria (PKU), 160
Phobias, cognitive therapy, 55–57
Physical abuse, 116–117
Physiotherapy, somatisation treatment, 100
Pilowsky's Illness Behaviour Questionnaire,
    93
Pimozide, 130
Plans, essay, 2, 9
Plasmid vectors, 144
Play therapy, 131
Police involvement, pathways to care, 219
Polymerase Chain Reaction (PCR), 145–146,
    158
Polymorphisms, 142
Population, ethnic group percentages, 215,
    216
Porphobilinogen deaminase gene, 151
Positive reinforcement, 124
Post-traumatic stress disorder (PTSD), 60–61
Post-viral fatigue syndrome *see* Chronic fatigue
    syndrome
Powell, Enoch, 187
Presenilin genes, 156
Prison
  lithium study, 172
  mental illness, 189, 198
Probes, 143, 144, 145
Problem-solving, 61–62
  personality disorders, 175
Procyclidine, 27
Propranolol, 35
Pseudodementia, 21
Psychodrama, 128

Psychodynamic therapy, child psychiatry
  group, 128
  individual, 130–131
Psychoeducational techniques
  child abuse, 122
  child pyschiatry, 127
Psychosis
  epidemiology, ethnic minority groups,
    211–212
  young people relapsing, 189
Psychosomatic family, 76
Psychosurgery, 20–21
Punishments, 126

Question expansion, 4–5
Questioning
  Socratic, 45
  triangular, 136–137
Questionnaires
  in diagnosis, transcultural psychiatry, 205
  illness behaviour, 93

Race, 201
Racial equality, 222–223
Racism, 207, 210
Reading, 1–2
Recombination fraction, 147
Referrals
  chronic fatigue syndrome, 108–109
  rehabilitation service, schizophrenia, 36
Reinforcing incompatible behaviour (RIB), 124
Relationships, somatisation, 99–100
Relaxation therapy, personality disorders, 175
Reprovision, 190–191
Resolvable problems, 62
Restriction enzymes, 142, 143, 144
Restriction Fragment Length Polymorphisms
  (RFLPs), 142
Reverse transcriptase, 145
Reversible Inhibitors of Monoamine Oxidase A
  (RIMA)
  treatment resistant depression, 16, 18
Risk assessment, child abuse, 120, 121
Risperidone, 34
Royal College of Psychiatrists
  care programme approach (CPA), 193–194
  community supervision order, 194
  Consensus statement, high dose neuroleptics,
    31–33
  Mental Health of the Nation document, 229
  staffing, old age psychiatry service, 231–
    232
  Ten-point plan and supervision registers,
    195–196
  training, racial equality, 222
Royal Free Disease *see* Chronic fatigue syndrome
Russell's sign, 68

Safety behaviours, 52, 55
Schemas/assumptions, 42
  dysfunctional, 43
  identifying, 50
Schizoaffective states, 150
Schizophrenia, 141, 149
  children, 130
  ethnic minority groups, 211–212
  genetic predisposition, 150–152
  reprovision exercise, 190–191
  treatment resistant, 25–40
    management, 26–28
    physical interventions, 29–35
    psychological interventions, 35–36
    social interventions, 36–38
Schizotypal personality disorder (SPD), 170
  individual psychotherapy, 176, 177
Schizotypy, 150
Schools of family therapy, 134–137
Section 136: 220
Selective serotonin reuptake inhibitors (SSRIs)
  personality disorders, 171–172
  somatisation, 101
  treatment resistant depression, 16, 17, 18
    and tricyclic combination, 19–20
Self-harm
  ethnic minority groups, 213
  personality disorders, 173, 174, 175
Self-induced vomiting, 68, 72, 75, 77
Serotonin, 16
Serotonin Noradrenaline Re-uptake Inhibitors
  (SNRIs), 16
Serotonin syndrome, 17, 19
Sertraline, 172
Sex chromosomes, pseudoautosomal region in
  schizophrenia, 152
Sexual abuse, 117
  associated psychiatric illnesses, 118
Shaping, behaviour therapy, 124
Sib pair analysis, 147, 150
Sick role, 92–93
  chronic fatigue syndrome, 109
  inmate, 186
  somatisation, 97
Single gene defects, 146, 149, 159
Sleep
  deprivation, 21
  problems in toddlers, 128
Social class
  ethnic minorities, 206
    The Black Report, 216–217
  illness behaviour, 91
Social skills training
  personality disorders, 175–176
  schizophrenia, 35
Socratic questioning, 45
Sodium valproate, 19

Somatic metaphor, 204
Somatic mutations, 142
Somatisation, 94–102
　aetiology, 96–97
　assessment and diagnosis, 95–96
　management, 97–102
　　by psychiatrist, 98–101
　　medication, 101
　　overall approach, 101–102
　with personality disorder, 178
　transcultural approaches, 204, 205
　see also Psychosomatic family
Somatisation disorder, 94, 104
Southern blotting, 143
Spectrum disorders, 150
Staff
　black and ethnic minority, 221–222
　old age psychiatry service, 231–232
Standards, setting in medical audit, 236
Starvation, 77
Stein and Test study, 191–192
Stimulation, lack of, 187
Strategic family therapy, 135–136
Stressors
　eating disorders, 75–76
　psychosocial, schizophrenia, 27–28,
　　36–37
Structural family therapy, 134–135
Structure
　essay, 3–5, 9
　MRCPsych exam, xi
Sub-caudate tractotomy, 21
Subcultural handicap, 159
Substance abuse
　dyssocial personality disorder, 178
　schizophrenia, 26–27
Successful community care, 189–190
Suicide rate
　ethnic minority groups, 213
　schizophrenia, 35
Supervision registers, 195, 196
　schizophrenia, 38
　see also Community supervision order
Systems theory, family therapy, 132

τ protein, 154
Tartrazine, 131
Team for the Assessment of Psychiatric Services
　(TAPS) Project, 190–191
Therapeutic community, 176
Thinking errors see Cognitive distortions

Thyroid hormones, 19
Tics, treatment of, 130
Total Institutions, 186–187
Tractotomy, sub-caudate, 21
Traditional healers, 205
Transcultural psychiatry, 201–227
　detecting disorders, 205
　epidemiology, 209–213
　illness behaviour, 91, 204–206
　management in, 214–223
　models of health and illness, 203
　transcultural factors causing illness, 206–209
Transcultural Special Interest Group, 201
Tranylcypromine, 171
Treatment resistant
　depression, 13–23
　schizophrenia, 25–26
Triangular questioning, 136–137
Tricyclic antidepressants
　Asian and Black patients, 215
　children, 128, 130
　chronic fatigue syndrome, 110–111
　personality disorders, 170–171
　somatisation, 101
　treatment resistant depression, 16, 17, 18
　　combined with MAOIs, 19
　　combined with SSRIs, 19–20
Trinucleotide repeat diseases, 157–158
Tube feeding, end stage anorexic patients,
　79–80
Tyrosine hydroxylase, 153

Vectors, DNA, 144
Velocardiofacial syndrome, 151–152
Venlafaxine, 16
Violent behaviour
　black patients, 220
　mentally ill in community, 192–193
Voluntary services, 189
　ethnic minority groups, 217–218
Vomiting, self-induced, 68, 72, 75, 77

Washout period, changing medication, 18
Weight, anorexia nervosa
　patient's control, 68
　working to increase, 77–79
Wing and Brown patient care study, 187
Wolpe, J, 57

Yeast artificial chromosomes (YACs), 144, 145,
　149